THE SHIATSU WAY TO HEALTH

THE SHIATSU WAY TO HEALTH

●　●　●

Relief and Vitality at a Touch

Toru Namikoshi

Translated by Kate McCandless
Illustrations by Joseph Cali

KODANSHA INTERNATIONAL
Tokyo and New York

jacket photography by Pamela Fernuik

distributed in the United States by Kodansha International/USA
Ltd., through Harper & Row, Publishers, Inc., 10 East 53rd Street,
New York, New York 10022.

published by Kodansha International Ltd., 2-2, Otowa
1-chome, Bunkyo-ku, Tokyo 112 and Kodansha Interna-
tional/USA Ltd., 10 East 53rd Street, New York, New York 10022.

first printing, 1988

ISBN 0-87011-796-3 (U.S.)
ISBN 4-7700-1296-9 (Japan)
LCC 87-81676

CONTENTS

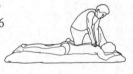

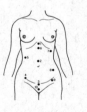
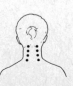

SHIATSU AND STRETCHING 107

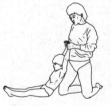

SHIATSU FOR CHILDREN 122

WHAT
IS
SHIATSU?

Shiatsu is a "hands on" method of preventive health care and therapy that increases vitality, relieves fatigue, and stimulates the body's natural healing power by pressure applied to key points on the body. In addition, it offers the warmth of a caring touch. This is particularly important now when medical care has become so highly technical and specialized and when our hectic urban lives have so many sources of stress, all of which take a toll on our bodies and minds. Even children often have busy schedules to keep and may suffer from physical and mental fatigue. Many people are anxious about the adverse effects of modern life on their health. There is no simple means to address their concern, but shiatsu offers a way to become aware of your body and to care for it—a way to take your health "into your own hands."

In this book, I have suggested ways in which you can use shiatsu on a daily basis to keep in touch with your own body. You don't have to drag through your days with a host of minor complaints (which only increase as you grow older). You can, with patience and discipline, improve your health, appearance, physical fitness, even sexual vigor. Furthermore, you can practice shiatsu with your friends and family, helping each other to a new physical awareness. Shiatsu is a wonderful way to give and receive caring without words and to share a few pleasant, relaxed moments in a busy day.

When we are in pain, or numb or sluggish, our instinctive response is to rub or press the area that bothers us. Even this simple action stimulates, to a degree, the natural functioning of the body systems. Applied systematically it will activate the body's natural healing power and restore the troubled area to normal. Though the natural response would be to stretch, rub, or scratch a particular area, most people today are more apt to try and ignore their discomfort or to take a pill.

Shiatsu treatment consists of pressure applied with the balls of the thumbs and fingers and the palms of the hands to specific points on the surface of the body. Traditionally, these points have been called *tsubo* in Japanese, which is the same word used for a jar or pot. The *tsubo* on the body tend to accumulate fatigue and stress. Pressing them brings relief, as early man discovered instinctively.

The ancient Chinese, through observation and experience, developed a system of diagnosis and treatment based on nearly seven hundred points on the body and the meridian lines of "energy flow" which connect them. One important method of treatment was acupuncture, in which needles were inserted at points along the meridians to correct the energy flow. This knowledge came to Japan over one thousand years ago, and in the eighteenth century, practitioners of traditional Japanese massage, or *anma*, incorporated this knowledge into their technique. In the 1920s, Tokujiro Namikoshi established shiatsu as a therapeutic system integrated with modern anatomy and physiology, coining the word *shiatsu*, literally "finger pressure," to describe his system.

The *tsubo* correspond to the muscles, bones, blood vessels, nerves, lymph vessels, and glands of the endocrine system that lie beneath them. Pressing these points not only stimulates the skin and relieves muscular stiffness, but regulates the nervous system, aids proper digestion, and stimulates blood and lymph circulation and hormonal secretion. Moreover, it both prevents disease and stimulates the body's natural recuperative power.

The essence of shiatsu lies in the use of the hands for both diagnosis and treatment. The sensitive fingertips can detect differences in temperature and stiffness, both indicators of the condition of the body. The type, degree, and duration of pressure is then adjusted to meet the specific needs of each area of the body and each individual. Because of this, shiatsu should be applied directly to the skin whenever possible.

Though the skills of a trained practitioner cannot be acquired overnight, this should not stop you from discovering for yourself how shiatsu works and becoming better acquainted with the human body. By giving regular shiatsu to yourself and others, you will grow sensitive to the needs of the body and begin to recognize the surface conditions signaling irregularities in the body. The essence of shiatsu lies not just in hands-on diagnosis and treatment, but in the warmth of another's touch. If the attitude of the giver of shiatsu is both careful and caring, and the attitude of the receiver is open and receptive, the experience is sure to be beneficial for both.

I have tried to emphasize procedures that increase stamina and vitality and ease common complaints, as well as to suggest ways to integrate shiatsu into your daily life. The basic techniques are given as clearly and concisely as possible, using a minimum of technical terms. I have supplemented these with a number of stretching exercises to increase the overall effectiveness. And I have included special chapters on shiatsu for children and improving one's appearance. My hope is that shiatsu will become an essential and enjoyable part of your daily life, that you will come to a deeper understanding of your body and its natural recuperative powers, and that shiatsu will serve you as well as it has served so many others.

Toru Namikoshi

BASIC
TECHNIQUES

The human hand, which most of us use so thoughtlessly, is actually a marvelous tool, a tool which has shaped human civilization. In modern times, with widespread automation, we use our hands very little; thus, practicing shiatsu is beneficial not only for health and well-being but for increasing manual dexterity and sensitivity.

Many sense receptors are located in the skin of the fingers, particularly in the fingertips and the palms. There are different types for sensing light touch, deep pressure, heat, cold, and pain. And although you may think your fingers all have the same degree of sensitivity, each has its specialty. The thumb is particularly sensitive to sharpness; the index finger can detect fine differences in texture, smoothness, or roughness; the middle finger can detect hardness and contour; and the ring finger is sensitive to heat.

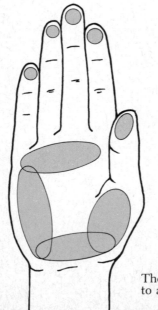

The areas of the hand used to apply pressure.

As you practice shiatsu, your hands will become more and more sensitive to slight variations in skin texture, temperature, and pliability, which will in turn enable you to adjust the degree and type of pressure, sense areas that need treatment, and give more and more effective shiatsu.

WAYS OF APPLYING PRESSURE

1. One thumb: Apply pressure with the ball of the thumb of either hand. Used for the sides of the neck, the Namikoshi point (page 18), and other locations.

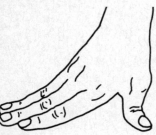

2. Two thumbs: Apply pressure with both thumbs, outer edges touching, with hands extended, fingers together. Used for the legs, back, and so on.

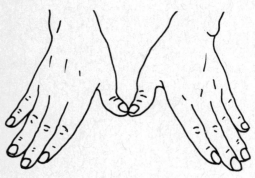

3. Overlapping thumbs: Place your left thumb over your right thumb and apply pressure with both simultaneously. Used for concentrated pressure to the first lateral shin point (page 19), the back of the legs, and other areas.

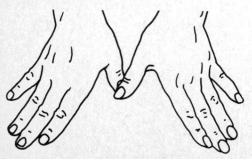

4. Three fingers: Apply pressure simultaneously with the index, middle, and ring fingers held close together for concentrated pressure on one point. Used for shoulders, chest, legs, and so forth.

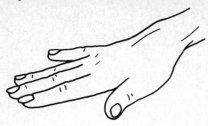

5. Three fingers (both hands): Apply three-finger pressure with both hands simultaneously, with the tips of the middle fingers touching. Sometimes this pressure is applied with the left fingers overlapping the right. Used for head, face, neck (sides and back), chest, abdomen, legs, and other areas.

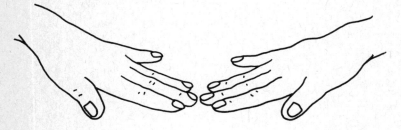

6. Overlapping middle fingers: Used particularly for concentrated pressure on the medulla oblongata (page 18). Place the ball of your right middle finger on the medulla oblongata. Then place the ball of your left middle finger on the nail of your right one and apply pressure.

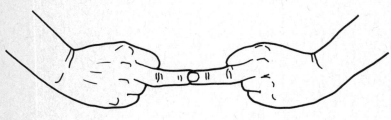

7. Overlapping middle and index fingers: Apply pressure with the ball of your index finger by crossing the ball of the middle finger of the same hand behind and placing it on the nail of the index finger. Used for the eye sockets, the sides of the nose, and between the shoulder blades.

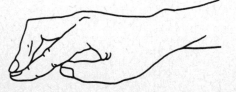

8. Opposing thumb and fingers: Apply pressure with the thumb and four fingers simultaneously, grasping the part to be worked on. Use for the nape of the neck and the calves.

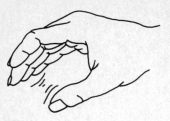

9. Palm: Apply pressure with the whole palm of the hand. For different areas you may use one palm, or two palms either side by side (with thumbs touching) or in separate positions. Used for the eyeballs, sides of the head, temples, chest, groin, and abdomen.

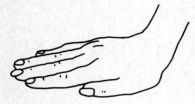

10. Overlapping palms: Place the left palm over the back of the right palm to stabilize it, and apply pressure with the right palm. Used for concentrated pressure to the chest and abdomen.

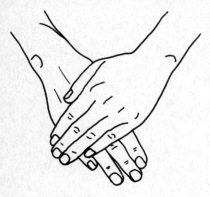

11. Clasped hands: Clasp your hands, interlocking the fingers, and apply pressure with the fleshy heels of the hands. Used for the kidney points.

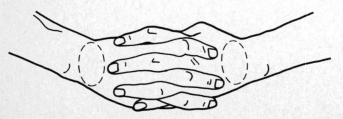

12. Base of the thumb: Apply pressure with the fleshy part of the palm at the base of the thumb.

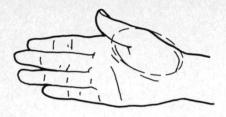

TYPES OF PRESSURE

1. Standard pressure: This is the type of pressure used most often. Apply pressure for about three seconds, then release gently.

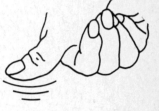

2. Sustained pressure: Mainly used with palm pressure. Maintain steady pressure for five to ten seconds. Do not apply strong pressure suddenly from the start, but increase the pressure gradually and steadily during the first few seconds.

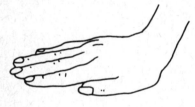

3. Graded pressure: Apply pressure to the same point in three stages of intensity. First, apply light pressure, then release without removing your hands from the body, then apply medium pressure, release, and apply strong pressure. Each application lasts from three to seven seconds.

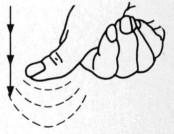

4. Vibrating pressure: Mainly used with palm pressure to stimulate the inner organs. Place your hand lightly on the skin and vibrate back and forth for five to ten seconds. These vibrations penetrate deeply and create a pleasant sensation.

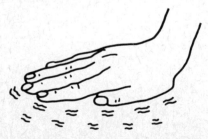

5. Flowing pressure: Move rhythmically and smoothly from point to point, pressing each point for about one second. Use for a long, continuous area of muscle stiffness.

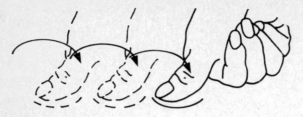

6. Palm stimulation: One palm, alternating palms, or overlapping palms may be used to stroke rapidly downward over the skin. Used for the back, abdomen, and chest.

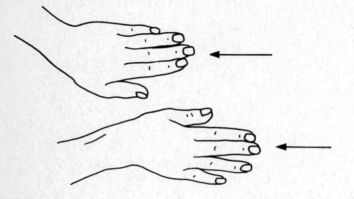

7. Suction pressure: Used mainly with palm pressure. Place the palm firmly against the skin and apply pressure by contracting and lifting up with the palm. This stretches the connective tissue between the skin and the muscles.

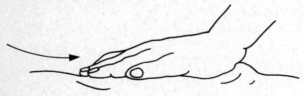

8. Circular pressure: Press the palm or palms firmly to the skin and move in a circular motion. The palm does not move over the skin. Used for the back, abdomen, and chest.

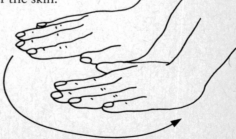

DEGREE OF PRESSURE

The degree of pressure depends on the degree of muscle stiffness in the area being treated. Giving abrupt, strong pressure to stiff muscles will not only be counter-effective but unpleasant. Strong pressure is best preceded by gentle pressure of short duration. With practice you will learn to observe changes in muscle condition and adjust the degree and type of pressure accordingly.

1. Touch: The hands barely touch the skin. Used to determine skin temperature and for infants.

2. Light pressure: Penetrates slightly through the skin into the connective tissues. Particularly good for small children and the elderly.

3. Standard pressure: Penetrates lightly through the skin to the surface of the muscles, producing a pleasurable sensation.

4. Medium pressure: Reaches deep into the muscles, producing a sensation of pleasurable discomfort.

5. Strong pressure: Used for working deep into stiff muscles. It may produce some pain, but only to the extent that your partner can tolerate it comfortably.

THE THREE TENETS OF SHIATSU

•*Shiatsu is suitable for everyone, from the very young to the very old.* For children, it helps to build a strong, resistant constitution. For adults, it helps maintain good health and a youthful appearance. For the elderly, it helps to keep the body resilient and to prevent the minor disorders brought on with aging. Even small children can learn to do self-shiatsu and to attend to the needs of their own bodies. And partner shiatsu is a way to share with friends and family the process of discovering true good health.

•*Shiatsu treats the body as a whole.* All the systems of the body are linked in complex mutual relationships. Shiatsu for a specific problem area is most effective when that area is given special attention as part of a whole-body treatment. When an area is treated in isolation the effects are more likely to be temporary.

•*Shiatsu is a way to give yourself a daily health check-up.* If you make shiatsu a regular habit, you will become aware of subtle changes in the condition of your body and be able to take early action to relieve fatigue, stress, or other minor problems. You may be surprised to realize how energized and positive you feel once you have incorporated shiatsu into your daily routine.

BASIC SHIATSU POINTS

The following five points are not only among the most fundamental points in shiatsu, but among the most important. They appear frequently in shiatsu procedures. As you come across them in giving shiatsu, the text will refer you to this page so that you can more readily locate the required point. With just a little practice, however, you will be able to find these vital points on your own.

■ Medulla Oblongata

Pressure to this point is essential in treating many ailments, including headaches, migraines, and hangovers. Unlike the first lateral forearm and shin points which require some practice before you will be able to pinpoint their location with ease and consistency, this point is easily found at the indentation at the top of the neck, just below the base of the skull. When you feel fatigued, pressing this point will bring a mild sense of relief. Medium to strong thumb pressure is standard.

■ Namikoshi Point

Named after the present author's father, this point is beneficial in treating diarrhea, menstrual problems, and other ailments in the region of the hips. A Namikoshi point may be found on either side of the buttocks over a nerve that branches out from the sciatic nerve, approximately 2 inches (at a slight diagonal) from the point where the pelvic bone protrudes at the hip. In general, strong thumb pressure is required.

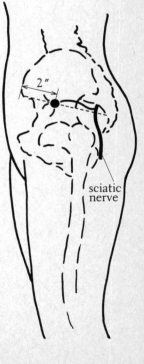

2"

sciatic nerve

■ First Lateral Forearm Point

This point, the first in a series of eight points that run along the outside of the lower arm from the elbow to the wrist, is located over a nerve and a muscle. Pressure applied here is effective in relieving tiredness in the arms. Like its companion point on the leg, when it is pressed you will experience a slight unpleasantness. This is natural but should serve to remind you to apply pressure judiciously: neither too strong nor too long, but gradually and with a steady hand.

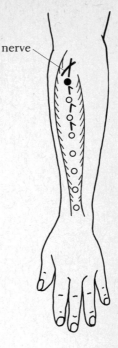

nerve

■ Solar Plexus

This abdominal point corresponds to the stomach and is thus instrumental in treating digestion, poor appetite in children, and other abdominal-related problems. The solar plexus points, numbers 1 and 6 of the 10-point abdominal series that appears throughout this volume, are located in the abdominal region directly below the rib cage. Use only palm pressure and apply as instructed.

■ First Lateral Shin Point

Attention given to this point, the first in a series of six points running along the outside of the lower leg, is instrumental in relieving leg fatigue. The point is directly above a nerve, which in turn stretches across a bone. When you experience a slight discomfort—the result of pressing the vein against the bone—you have found the point. Since a nerve is being pressed, apply pressure gradually, neither too strong nor too long.

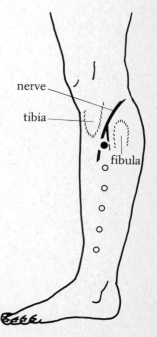

nerve

tibia

fibula

BEFORE YOU BEGIN

Before beginning, make sure your hands are clean and your fingernails are cut.

Take a few minutes to breathe deeply, calm yourself, and clear your mind of distractions.

To ensure that the shiatsu you give is even, rhythmical, and pleasant, coordinate your breathing with your movements, exhaling as you press; maintain correct, comfortable posture; and concentrate on what you are doing.

Encourage your partner to breathe naturally and regularly, exhaling when you press.

Press only with the palms of the hands and the balls of the fingers and thumbs, not the fingertips or the joints.

Finally, use the correct pressure points and procedures. Do not hurry or try to perform miracles. Patience and regularity give the best results.

A FEW CAUTIONS

Shiatsu is a safe, rejuvenating activity. But as with most such physical therapies, a few common-sense guidelines should be followed:

1. Do not press any one point for too long or make any one session too long.

2. Always consider the age and condition of your partner.

3. Do not make someone with a painful condition that limits mobility lie or sit in an uncomfortable position.

Avoid giving shiatsu:

1. When the stomach is empty or too full. Wait at least thirty minutes after a meal.

2. In cases of extreme weakness or exhaustion.

3. In cases of infectious disease, including infectious skin disease, high fever, or acute inflammation.

4. In cases of stomach ulcer or other ailments of the internal organs which require professional medical care.

FULL-BODY
SHIATSU

A complete shiatsu session is as bracing as a well-given massage and much more therapeutic. By following the step-by-step directions here, you can give full-body shiatsu to a partner or to yourself. In total it takes about ninety minutes. However, in the beginning a single session should last no longer than forty to sixty minutes, so choose a section or two of the body to concentrate on each time until you have learned the points and procedure. Most of the basic sequences appear in this section. Once you have become familiar with them treating separate parts of the body for such ailments as headaches and insomnia becomes little more than applying what is presented here.

Full-body partner shiatsu begins with your partner lying on his or her right side. The left side of the neck and back is pressed, then your partner shifts over onto his or her left side and the sequence is repeated. Next, shiatsu is given to the back of the body from head to toe. A short exercise to adjust the back completes the second stage. The final stage—shiatsu to the front of the body—finishes with a thorough treatment to the abdominal area, perhaps the most vital area of all.

These directions are for working on a padded floor, though any firm and comfortable surface, including a massage table, will do. A Japanese futon or thick blanket folded and spread over a carpet works well. Use a thin pillow or folded towel to support the head. If the room is at all cool, cover your partner with a light blanket and uncover only the part of the body you are working on.

Shiatsu for the head, neck, shoulders, and upper back can be conveniently performed with your partner kneeling on the floor or sitting on a stool. This will allow you more freedom of motion and give more leverage for applying certain kinds of pressure.

Directions are given for the left side, but always repeat the shiatsu for the right side of whatever area you are working on. Where not otherwise indicated, you should use standard pressure (page 14) for about three seconds per application. At the end of a session, encourage your partner to rest for at least ten minutes, preferably longer.

Side of the Body

NECK

Full-body shiatsu begins with the neck and ends with the abdominal region—the most important, as well as the most difficult, areas of the body to give shiatsu to. The neck muscles
support the head, so they are particularly vulnerable to tension.
Stiffness in these muscles puts pressure on the important blood
vessels, nerves, and glands in the neck area and impedes their
functioning.

The first point on each side of the front of the neck is a vital
pulse point on the carotid artery, which regulates blood pressure,
heartbeat, and blood supply to the brain. The vagus nerve, which
regulates the internal organs, parallels the carotid artery. Between the fourth points on the front of the neck is the thyroid
gland. Thus, shiatsu to the front of the neck is beneficial for
a great number of ailments, including high blood pressure,
digestive disorders, and respiratory diseases. Shiatsu to the sides
of the neck is particularly helpful for motion sickness, dizziness,
and ear ailments. Shiatsu to the back of the neck is good for
insomnia, headache, and sinusitis.

Be very careful not to press too hard when giving shiatsu to
the neck. Gauge the degree of tension in the muscles and give
gradual, gentle pressure.

1. Have your partner lie on her right side with both arms forward
in a natural position, her right leg extended and her left leg bent.
Kneel behind your partner on your left knee, with your right knee
raised. Make a stable three-point base by putting your left hand
on the floor in front of your partner.

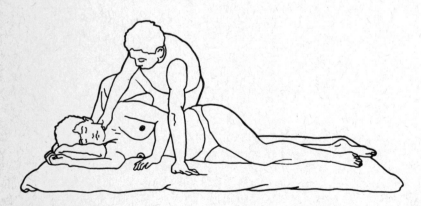

Place your right thumb gently under your partner's jaw. You will
feel a pulse where the carotid artery passes near the surface. Using
this as your starting point, apply pressure gently for two seconds
to each of the points along the left front of the neck. Repeat twice.

SELF-SHIATSU: Sit or kneel in a comfortable position. Use your left thumb for the left side, your right thumb for the right. Press gently for three seconds, first one side, then the other. (Do not press both sides at once.)

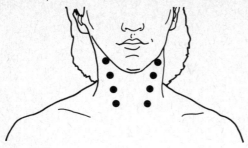

2. Have your partner lean slightly forward, so that the side of the neck faces directly upward. Apply slightly stronger pressure with two thumbs (or overlapping thumbs) for two seconds to the points beginning just below the bony extension of the skull behind the the earlobe. Repeat twice.

SELF-SHIATSU: Use three-finger pressure on both sides at once.

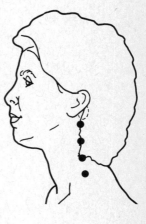

3. Have your partner lean farther forward again, so that the back of the neck faces upward. Apply two-thumb (or overlapping-thumb) pressure to the points on the left back side of the neck. You may press a bit more strongly here. However, be careful not to press on the vertebrae at the fourth point, but press closer to the shoulder. Repeat twice.

SELF-SHIATSU: Use three-finger pressure on both sides at once. Press in the direction of the tip of your nose.

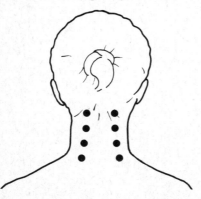

NOTE: At this point, if you are doing partner shiatsu, repeat the same sequence for the right side. However, if you are also doing the "optional sequence," wait until you have finished that before giving shiatsu to the right side.

OPTIONAL SEQUENCE

The following five steps can be done while your partner is still on her side, as a prelude to the full treatment to the back of the body. Although the points are pressed again in the following section, the angle is different, so the steps below are efficacious in their own right.

Treating the back of the body from this position is particularly good for a pregnant woman or anyone who is not comfortable when lying on his or her stomach.

1. Holding the forehead with your left hand, apply medium to strong thumb pressure to the medulla oblongata (page 18) with your right thumb. Repeat twice.

2. Move so that you are kneeling at the top of your partner's head with your left knee raised. Extend your arms and, supporting the shoulder with your fingers, apply overlapping-thumb pressure (right over left) to the upper shoulder point at the base of the neck in line with the points on the side of the neck. Press for five seconds. Repeat twice.

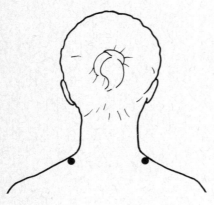

3. Move so that you are kneeling facing your partner's shoulder-blade area. Apply overlapping-thumb pressure to the points between the left shoulder blade and the spine, taking care not to press the bone.

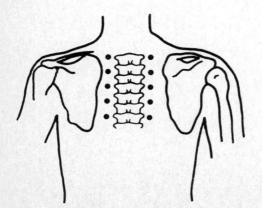

4. Move so that your are kneeling beside your partner's buttocks with your right knee raised. Apply overlapping-thumb pressure to the ten points down the left side of the spine, starting with the fifth upper-back point (of the previous step).

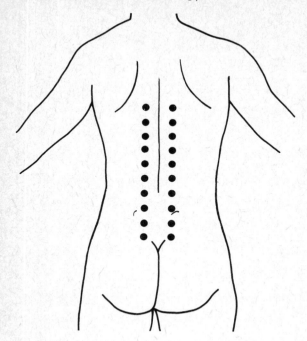

5. Place your left hand on your partner's left hip. With your right hand, apply palm pressure to four points down the left side of the back. Repeat twice, then rapidly stroke the left side of the spine twice.

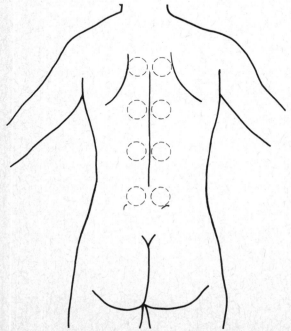

Back of the Body

HEAD, NECK, AND SHOULDERS

Shiatsu to the back of the body is given with your partner in a prone position. It begins with the points on the head, neck, and upper shoulders. However, when you are limited by considerations of time or space, or dealing with a specific problem, such as headache, this area may easily be treated with your partner in a sitting position.

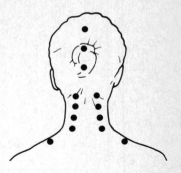

1. Have your partner lie facedown with arms pointing out and bent upward at the elbow, or with hands under her head. The chest rests flat on the floor, the legs are extended. Support your partner's forehead with a low pillow or folded towel.

Kneel at your partner's left side with your left knee raised. Apply two-thumb pressure to the points down the back of the head. These points reach only to the highest point on the *back* of the head. Repeat twice.

SELF-SHIATSU: Remain in a sitting or kneeling position. Use three-finger pressure with both hands.

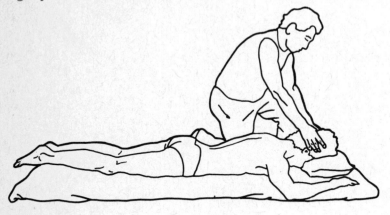

2. Apply medium to strong overlapping-thumb pressure for five seconds to the medulla oblongata (page 18). Repeat twice. This point affects the pituitary gland.

SELF-SHIATSU: Use overlapping-middle-finger pressure (left over right) and slowly tilt your head back slightly until the pressure penetrates.

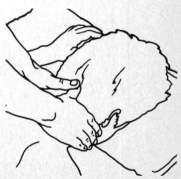

3. Support the crown of the head with your left hand, and use the opposed thumb and four fingers to press the four points on each side of the back of the neck. Repeat twice.

SELF-SHIATSU: Use three-finger pressure on both sides at once. Press in the direction of the tip of your nose.

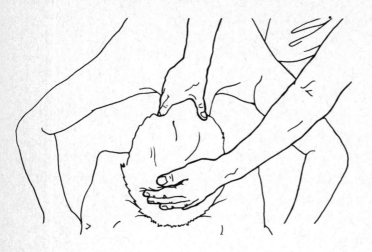

4. Have your partner remove the pillow and turn her face toward the side to receive shiatsu. Kneel just beyond your partner's head, facing her at a slight angle. Brace yourself with your right hand on the floor. With your left thumb, press the upper-shoulder point at the base of the neck for five seconds. Press in the direction of the center of the torso, at the level of the solar plexus. Repeat twice.

SELF-SHIATSU: Apply three-finger pressure with your right hand to your left upper shoulder. If your shoulders are particularly stiff, you may want to use vibrating pressure. Repeat for the right shoulder.

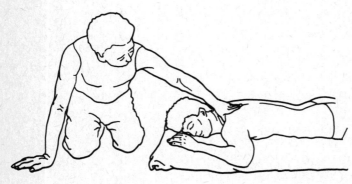

BACK

The upper back can only be reached with the help of a partner. Like the neck, it is particularly susceptible to stiffness and tension, because the muscles between the backbone and the shoulder blades are closely layered. People who work with their arms in one position for a lengthy period often have trouble with upper-back stiffness.

The points on the left side of the upper back affect the bronchia, lungs, heart, and stomach, and those on the right side, the bronchia, lungs, liver, and gallbladder. The fourth and fifth lower-back points affect the kidneys; the ninth and tenth, the sciatic nerve and the intestines.

When treating the back, kneel with your upper body erect and your arms fully extended. Press with the balls of your thumbs, gradually and steadily, to release muscle tension. The relaxing effect will penetrate through the muscle layers near the surface to the deeper layers. If you push too vigorously or abruptly when there is stiffness, the muscles will only tense more in reaction. Also, be careful not to press directly with your thumbs on the shoulder blades, backbone, or ribs.

1. Kneel at your partner's side, with your knee raised. Apply overlapping-thumb pressure for two seconds to the points between the left shoulder blade and the spine. Repeat twice.

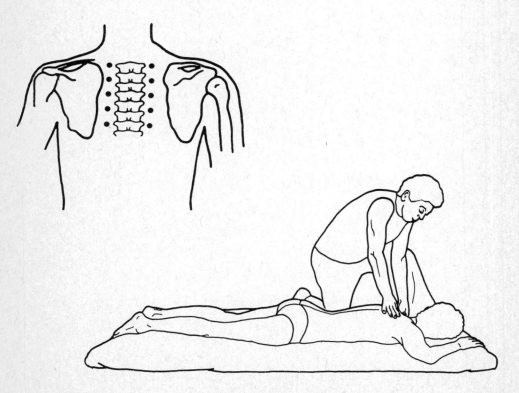

2. Apply overlapping-thumb pressure for two seconds to each of the ten points along the left side of the spine, beginning with the point level with the lower edge of the left shoulder blade (this point is the same as the fifth upper-back point) and work down to the pelvic bone. Repeat twice.

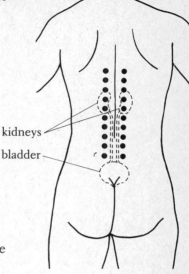

kidneys

bladder

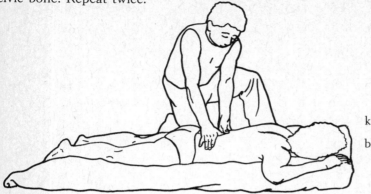

SELF-SHIATSU

1. Apply medium pressure with your thumbs to both sides of the lower back at once.

2. Clasp your hands behind your back so that the heels of your hands can press the fourth and fifth points over the kidneys. First, apply standard pressure for three seconds, then apply vibrating pressure for ten seconds.

HIP AREA

When pressing the sacrum, or tailbone, you are really working on the muscles attached to it. Be sure to use gradual, steady pressure. The sacral points are related to sexual vitality. The points on the buttocks are good for gynecological ailments. The Namikoshi points have long been known as a key to the treatment of diarrhea, sciatic pain, menstrual irregularity, and other ailments.

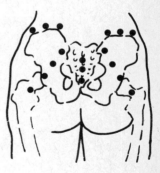

1. Apply overlapping-thumb pressure to the points along the upper edge of the hipbone, working outward. Repeat twice.

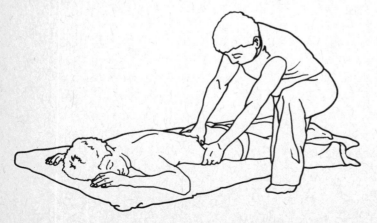

2. Apply two-thumb pressure to the three points on the tailbone. Repeat twice.

3. Apply overlapping-thumb pressure to the points on the buttocks, starting with the point to the left of the upper-tailbone point and working diagonally toward the hip joint. Repeat twice.

4. Shift your position so that you are kneeling facing your partner's hips. Locate the Namikoshi point (page 18). Use a strong kneading pressure with overlapping thumbs, steadily increasing for five seconds, then gently release. Repeat twice.

SELF-SHIATSU: Press the points in steps 1 through 3 while standing or kneeling. Use your thumbs to apply pressure to both sides at once. Press the Namikoshi points with an upward kneading motion.

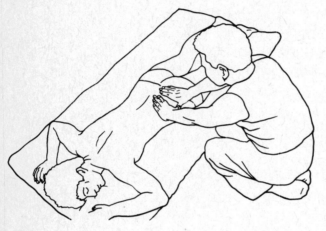

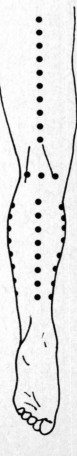

LEGS

When the leg muscles are stiff, blood circulation is poor and the legs chill and tire easily. Poor circulation also leads to swelling and varicose veins. Those who work standing or sitting continuously are particularly prone to poor circulation. Shiatsu will increase the suppleness of the muscles and improve circulation. Muscles can be very sensitive when stiff, so work carefully, adjusting the pressure according to stiffness and your partner's response.

1. Kneel at your partner's left side with your left knee raised. Apply overlapping-thumb pressure to the ten points on the back of the thigh, starting at the point just beneath the buttock. Repeat twice.

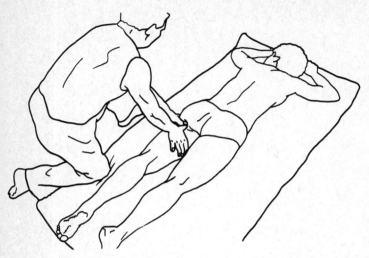

2. Apply two-thumb pressure to the points on the back of the knee, working from the inside out. Repeat twice.

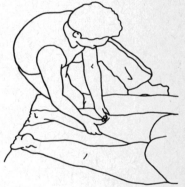

3. Apply two-thumb pressure to the eight points running down the center of the calf, working toward the foot. Repeat twice.

SELF-SHIATSU: Sit on a comfortable surface or in a chair with legs extended. Bend your left leg and apply three-finger pressure with both hands to the points on the back of the thigh. Then extend your leg and press the back of the knee, and bend it again for the calf.

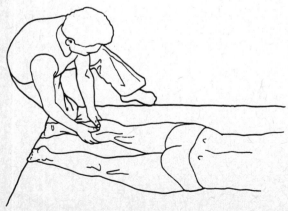

4. Shift so that you are kneeling facing your partner's calf. Press the six points on the outer side of the calf from the knee to the Achilles tendon by grasping the calf with both hands, thumbs together. Repeat twice.

SELF-SHIATSU: Bend your left leg inward so that it rests on or crosses over your right leg. Apply overlapping-thumb pressure to the points on the outer side of the calf.

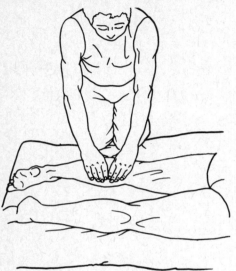

FEET

Shiatsu to the feet should be given frequently to relieve fatigue and promote relaxation. For those whose feet chill easily, or who have weak kidneys or digestive ailments, give special attention to the sole of the foot, particularly the arch.

1. Kneel alongside your partner's calf, facing the feet. Wrap both hands around the ankle and lift the foot slightly. Apply kneading pressure with both thumbs to the three points along the base of the Achilles tendon. Repeat twice.

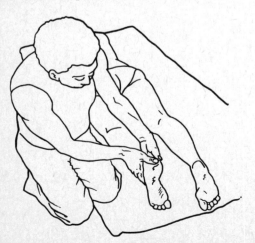

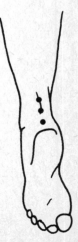

2. Lower the foot and rest your fingers on the sole of the foot. Press the points on both sides of the heel with your thumbs at the same time, moving from the heel toward the toes. Repeat twice.

SELF-SHIATSU: Support the foot with your left hand over the instep, and press the above points with opposing thumb and three fingers of your right hand.

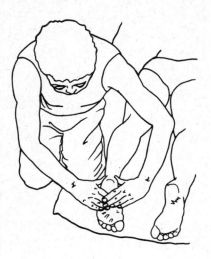

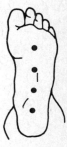

3. Raise your right knee and extend your arms. Apply two-thumb pressure to the points on the sole of the foot, from toes to heel. Repeat twice.

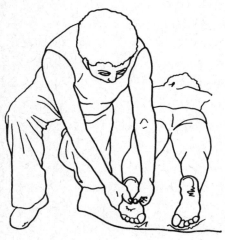

4. Finally, apply deep pressure with overlapping thumbs to the arch (the third point on the sole). Repeat twice.

SELF-SHIATSU: Use overlapping thumbs to press the points on the sole.

NOTE: For partner shiatsu, repeat the sequence for the back of the body on the right side. Again, for self-shiatsu, you should be doing both sides as you go, either simultaneously or first the left then the right side.

ADJUSTING THE BACK (PARTNER SHIATSU ONLY)

In partner shiatsu, after finishing both the left and right sides from shoulder to foot, you may follow this procedure for adjusting the back. This will correct irregularities in the alignment of the spinal column and relieve pressure on the spinal nerves and muscles.

1. Kneel at your partner's right side so that you can reach the upper back, with your right knee and hips raised. Place your left palm on the left shoulder blade and your right palm on the right shoulder blade. Apply counterclockwise circular pressure with your left palm three times, then clockwise circular pressure with your right palm three times; repeat both actions simultaneously five times.

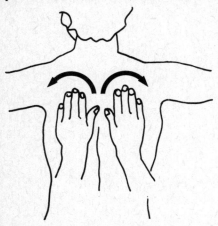

2. Move back slightly. Place both palms on the sides of the torso at the level of the diaphragm, with the thumbs below the shoulder blades. Coordinating your movements with your breathing, push upward and then downward rhythmically. Hands should not slide over surface of the skin, but should "pull" the skin with them as they move up and down. Do ten times.

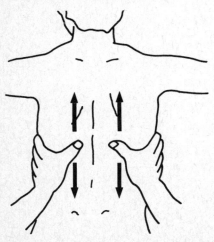

3. Apply circular palm pressure to the buttocks as you did to the shoulder blades in step 1.

4. Shift so that you are kneeling facing your partner's back. Place both palms crosswise over the top of the spine as shown. Raise your hips slightly and have your partner exhale as you push and then pull. Do this twice. As before, hands "pull" the skin with them. Start at the top and work down the spine in six steps. Repeat once.

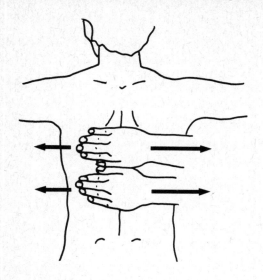

5. Again kneel with your right knee and hips raised. Place your left palm at the top of the back over the spine, with fingers pointing toward the head. Place your right palm over your left at a right angle. Press down the spine in six steps. Pressure should be steady and synchronized with your partner's breathing. Repeat once.

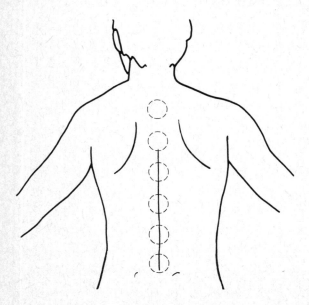

6. Place both palms over the spine at the top of the back, right over left, with fingers pointing toward the head. Stroke quickly and smoothly down the spine to the tailbone. Repeat twice.

Front of the Body

LEGS

After having received shiatsu to the sides and back of the body, your partner will be much more relaxed and able to benefit from shiatsu to the front of the body, especially the very important abdominal area.

Shiatsu to the front of the legs, as to the back, improves circulation and is good for tiredness, pain, swelling, or numbness in the legs, as well as high blood pressure, dizziness, digestive ailments, and menstrual pain.

1. Have your partner lie on her back with legs extended. Support the head with a thin pillow or folded towel and, if you wish, drape a cloth over your partner's eyes to shield them from the light and allow complete relaxation. Kneel at your partner's left side with your right knee raised. Place your left hand on the lower part of your partner's left thigh for support. With your right hand, apply palm pressure to the groin point for five seconds. Repeat twice.

SELF-SHIATSU: Lie on your back and apply three-finger pressure to the center of the groin.

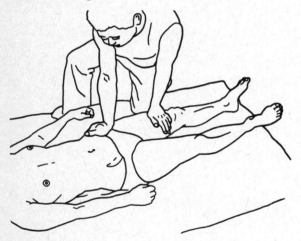

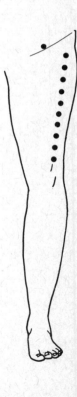

2. Apply overlapping-thumb pressure to the ten points along the front of the thigh, working toward the knee. Repeat twice.

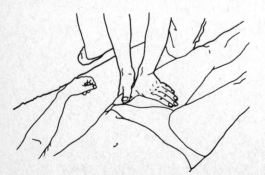

3. Have your partner turn her left knee outward at about a forty-five-degree angle. Apply overlapping-thumb pressure to the ten points along the inside of the thigh. Repeat twice.

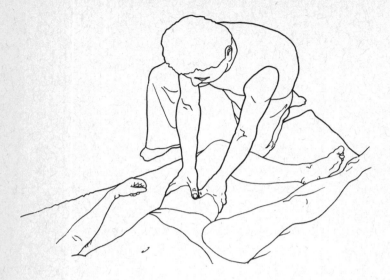

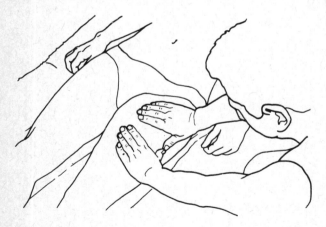

4. Have your partner extend her leg. Kneel facing the thigh and apply two-thumb pressure to the ten points along the outside of the thigh from the base of the thigh to the knee. Repeat twice.

SELF-SHIATSU: Remain sitting on the floor with legs extended. Apply two-thumb pressure to the top of the thigh, then turn the leg outward to press the inside of the thigh. Finally, turn the leg inward and press the points at the side.

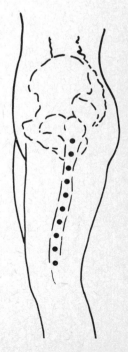

5. Kneel facing the knee and frame the kneecap with your hands. Press the points around the bottom of the kneecap with the left thumb, then press the points around the top of the kneecap with the right thumb. Repeat twice.

SELF-SHIATSU: Raise your knee slightly and wrap your fingers around the back of the knee for support. Apply two-thumb pressure to the points around the bottom of the kneecap, then those around the top of the kneecap, working inward.

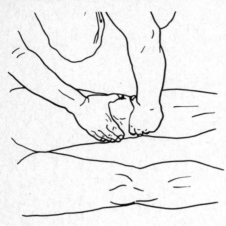

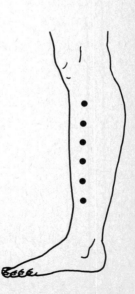

6. Find the first lateral shin point (page 19). It is located over a nerve, so pressure should be gradual. Apply fairly strong pressure with overlapping thumbs. Repeat twice. Pressing this point is particularly effective for relieving leg fatigue.

7. Move so that you are facing the calf. Using the fingers of both hands to grip the inside of the shinbone, apply pressure with overlapping thumbs to the points on the outside of the calf, from the first lateral shin point to the ankle. Repeat twice.

SELF-SHIATSU: Bend your knee inward so that it rests on your right leg. Apply overlapping-thumb pressure to the first shin point, then the remaining five points along the outside of the calf.

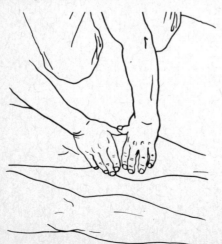

FEET

Shiatsu to the feet is particularly good for stimulating blood circulation and relieving fatigue.

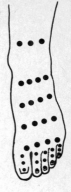

1. Kneel beside the calf, facing the feet. Cup the toes of the left foot with your left hand and, with your right thumb, press the three points across the front of the ankle, working inward. Repeat twice.

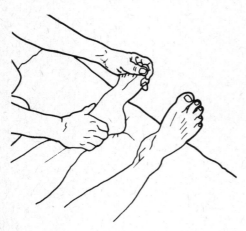

2. Still supporting the foot, apply pressure with your right thumb to each of the four rows running across the foot. Start with the row at the base of the toes and the point between the big and second toes and work outward. Points are located between the bones of the instep.

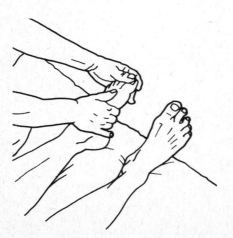

3. Shift to face your partner's left ankle. Steady the left ankle with your right hand and, with your left thumb and index finger, apply pressure to the points on the top and bottom of each toe. Start at the base of each toe and work from the big toe to the little toe, pulling gently as you press.

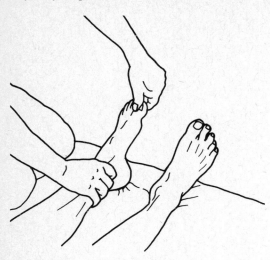

4. Still steadying the ankle with your right hand, wrap your left hand lightly around the toes and bend them rapidly back and forth several times. Repeat the same bending motion once on the upper portion of the foot.

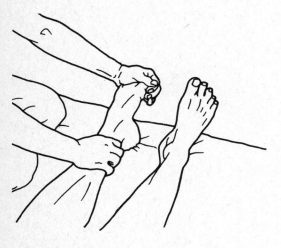

5. Finally, kneel facing the soles of your partner's feet. Brace your partner's right foot against your left knee. Grasp your partner's left leg near the ankle with both hands and raise the foot about four inches higher than your own knee. Pull firmly for three seconds, then gently lower it.

SELF-SHIATSU: Use two-thumb pressure for the points across the front of the ankle. Then follow steps 2 through 4, pressing the feet and toes the same as you would for partner shiatsu.

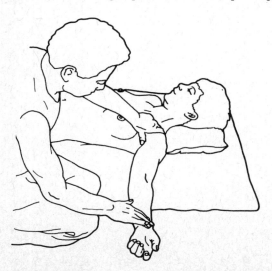

ARMS

Shiatsu to the arms is good for pain, numbness, chill, or shaking. Those concerned about heart disease should give special attention to the left arm (see also Strengthening the Heart, page 57). When giving shiatsu to someone with bursitis, do not force the arms into painful positions.

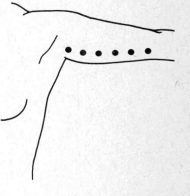

1. Have your partner lie on her back, her left arm outstretched. Kneel at your partner's left side, facing the arm. Place the three middle fingers of your right hand on the wrist pulse. Search for the pulse point in the armpit with your left thumb. When you think you have found it, press, and if you have located the correct spot, the pulse in the wrist will temporarily stop. Place your right thumb over your left thumb and apply medium pressure for five seconds. Repeat twice.

SELF-SHIATSU: Use three-finger pressure for the pulse point.

2. Apply two-thumb pressure to each of the six points on the inside of the upper arm, starting from the pulse in the armpit. Repeat twice.

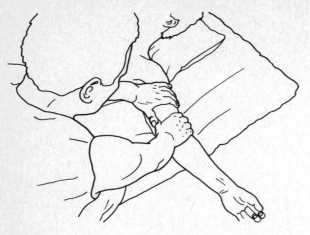

3. Move your partner's arm down to a forty-five-degree angle, and kneel with one knee on each side of the hand. Apply two-thumb pressure to the points on the underside of the elbow, working inward.

4. Apply overlapping-thumb pressure first to the eight points on the inside of the lower arm from the elbow to the wrist on the little-finger side. Repeat with the middle and third rows. Use a slight pulling motion in the direction of the wrist.

SELF-SHIATSU: Apply thumb pressure to the points in steps 2 through 4.

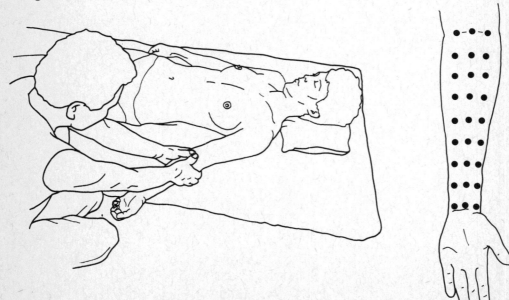

5. Kneel facing your partner's shoulder and raise your hips so that you are looking directly down at the shoulder. Apply overlapping-thumb pressure to the points along the groove where the arm joins the body, starting with the uppermost point. Repeat twice.

SELF-SHIATSU: Apply thumb pressure to the points while loosely gripping your shoulder with the fingers of the same hand.

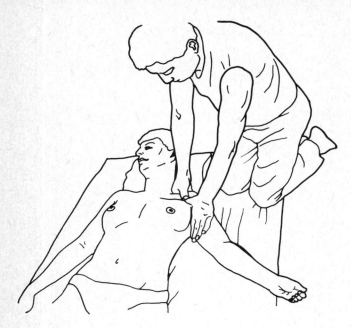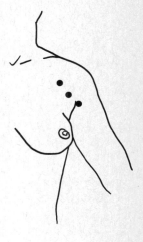

6. Shift so that you are facing the upper arm. Apply two-thumb pressure to the points along the outside of the upper arm, from the shoulder to the elbow. Repeat twice.

SELF-SHIATSU: Apply three-finger pressure to the points along the outside of the upper arm.

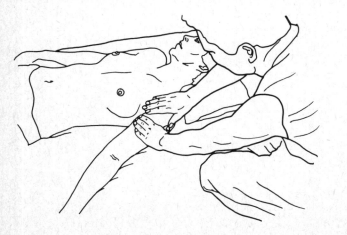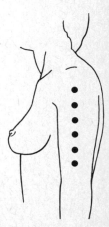

7. Move so that you are kneeling beside your partner's hip, facing the head. Have your partner place his left hand on your left knee. Apply overlapping-thumb pressure to each of the eight points on the outside of the lower arm from the elbow joint to the wrist. (The first of these points is the first lateral forearm point on the arm. Like the first lateral shin point on the leg, it is located over a nerve and is particularly effective for relieving fatigue.) Repeat twice.

SELF-SHIATSU: Apply thumb pressure to the points along the outside of the lower arm.

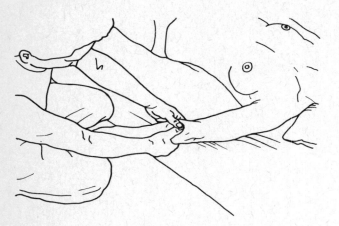

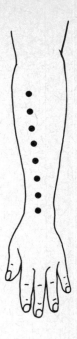

HANDS

Shiatsu to the hands improves circulation and stimulates the connection between the hands and the brain.

1. Hold your partner's left hand palm-down as shown, curling your fingers under to support the hand. Apply pressure with your thumbs, first to the two outside rows, then to the two inside. The rows run between the long bones of the hand, which correspond to each finger.

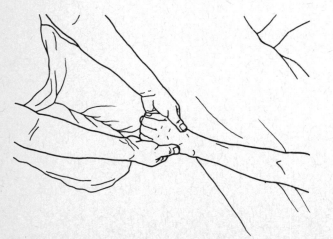

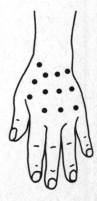

2. Shift your partner's hand to your right hand. Using your left thumb and index finger, apply pressure to the points on the top and bottom of the thumb and then the points on the sides, working from base to tip and pulling as you press. Follow the same procedure for the fingers. After doing the middle finger, apply pressure with the other hand.

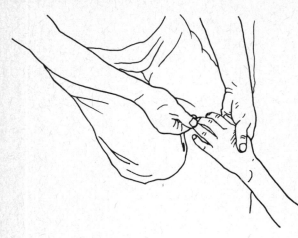

3. Turn the hand palm-up and apply two-thumb pressure to the points down center of the palm, working toward the fingers. Repeat twice. Then press the center point strongly with overlapping thumbs.

SELF-SHIATSU: Apply thumb pressure to all the hand and finger points in steps 1 through 3. Use thumb pressure for the palm points.

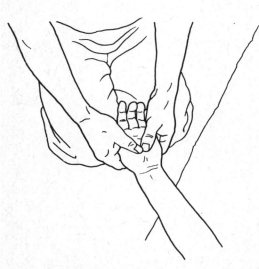

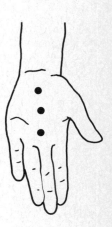

4. In the same position, raise the arm slightly, lean back, and pull the arm, then release.

5. Finally, stand up and, with both hands, lift your partner's lower arm near the wrist until it is at a ninety-degree-angle with the floor. Hold the wrist in your right hand and, with your left hand, bend over and stroke the upper arm from armpit to elbow, stepping away and bringing the arm back as you do so. Repeat twice, then pull the arm gently from its almost horizontal position.

Return the arm to the ninety-degree position, grab the lower arm, and gently pull it straight up for two seconds. Release and let the arm fall to the side.

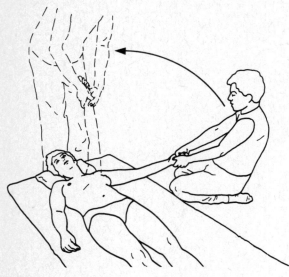

HEAD

Shiatsu to the head is effective for headache, migraine, mental fatigue, and, somewhat more surprisingly, insomnia. Improving circulation in the brain, it helps prevent memory loss and "dullness." It also stimulates the scalp and promotes healthier hair.

1. Before giving shiatsu to the head, you may want to cover the hair with a light cotton cloth. Kneel behind your partner, facing the head. Place the tips of both thumbs together on the median line of the head at the hairline of the forehead. Apply overlapping-thumb pressure to the points along this line to the crown of the head. Repeat twice.

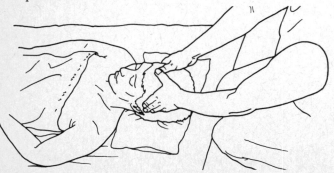

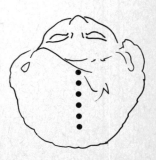

2. Steady the right side of the head lightly with your right hand and, starting at the crown of the head, apply thumb pressure to the six rows of three points each on the left side of the head. Work from the median line outward, finishing at the hairline. Repeat for the right side of the head.

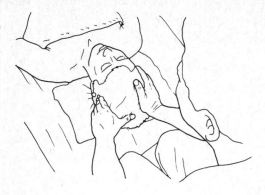 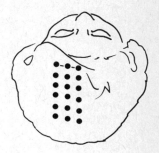

3. Again apply pressure to the six points along the median line from the hairline to the crown of the head.

4. Use both thumbs to apply pressure to the six rows of points on each side simultaneously, from the crown to the hairline, working outward from the median line.

5. Finally, work down the median line again from the hairline and, at the last point on the crown of the head, slowly increase the pressure, then gently release.

SELF-SHIATSU: Follow the same procedure as above, using three-finger pressure, but skipping steps 2 and 3. Then apply palm pressure to the sides of the head for five to ten seconds. Repeat twice.

FACE

More than any other part of the body, the face mirrors our state of health. In traditional oriental physiognomy, the forehead is called the "garden of heaven"; when the forehead has a poor color, the person's fate is sure to take a turn for the worse. By giving shiatsu to the forehead, you will improve your partner's color, and perhaps her fate as well. Also, the lowest forehead point is particularly good for sinus trouble. Shiatsu to the nose points also brings relief of congestion and can help to reduce swelling and restore the appearance of the nose after operations for sinusitis or nasal polyps.

Shiatsu for the eyes relieves eyestrain and can help vision problems. Pressing the gums through the skin around the mouth improves dental health and keeps the skin pliant. Overall, regular shiatsu to the face will help keep the skin smooth, moist, and supple. (See also Skin Care, page 100.)

1. Kneel behind your partner's head with your hips raised. Apply overlapping-thumb pressure to the forehead points, beginning with the point between the eyebrows. Repeat twice.

SELF-SHIATSU: Use three-finger pressure with both hands.

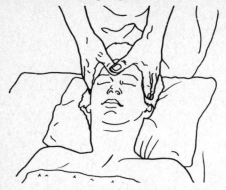

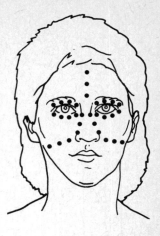

2. Lower your hips. Apply overlapping middle/index-finger pressure to both sides of the nose simultaneously from top to bottom. The first set of points is slightly below the inner edge of the eyes at the base of the nose, the second slightly lower on each side of the nasal bone, and the last on each side of the nostrils.

SELF-SHIATSU: Apply pressure to both sides with overlapping middle and index fingers.

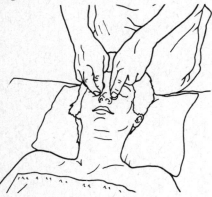

3. Apply three-finger pressure to the points located along the lower edge of each cheekbone, doing both sides simultaneously.

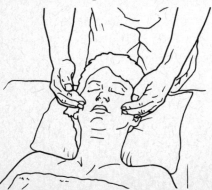

4. Place the right hand lightly on the forehead to steady the head and, with the left thumb, apply pressure to the four points along the lower edge of the left eye socket, from the inner edge to the outer edge of the eye, then to the four points along the upper edge.

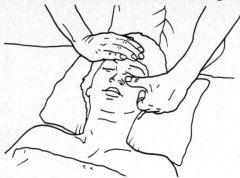

5. Next, press the three left temple points. Repeat the same procedure for the points around the right eye, changing hands.

SELF-SHIATSU: Use three-finger pressure for points in steps 3 through 5, pressing both sides at once.

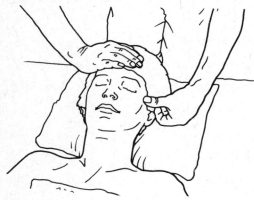

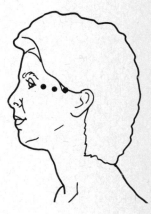

6. Place the fingers over the eyes, fingertips touching. Apply very light pressure to both eyeballs for ten seconds, then release gently. If your partner is wearing contact lenses, omit this procedure.

SELF-SHIATSU: Place the palms over the eyes and follow the same procedure as above.

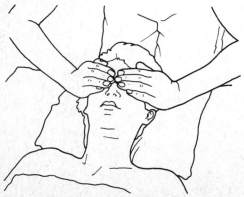

CHEST

Shiatsu releases tension in the chest muscles, making breathing deeper and easier. It is effective against asthma, heartburn, and nerve pain in the chest.

1. Kneel behind your partner's head and rest your right hand lightly on the right side of your partner's chest. With your left thumb, apply pressure for two seconds to points between the left ribs, starting from the point nearest the breastbone and working outward. After doing the left side, repeat on the right side. If your partner is a woman, work around the breasts.

SELF-SHIATSU: Press both sides at once, using three fingers spread to press three rows at a time.

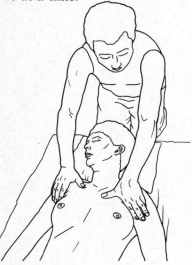

2. Apply two-thumb pressure to the five points along the breastbone, working downward. Do not press on the lower, cartilaginous part of the breastbone. Repeat twice.

SELF-SHIATSU: Use three-finger pressure with both hands.

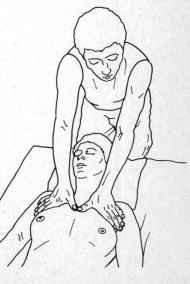

3. For men, place both hands firmly on the chest and move in a circular motion, clockwise with the right and counterclockwise with the left. Complete ten circles. For women, apply circular pressure to the chest area above the breasts.

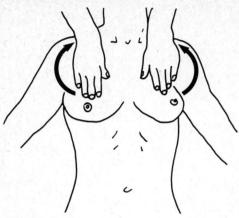

4. Then place both palms on the upper chest and stroke downward as your partner exhales. For women, stroke the upper chest area only. Repeat once.

SELF-SHIATSU: Follow the same procedure for steps 3 and 4.

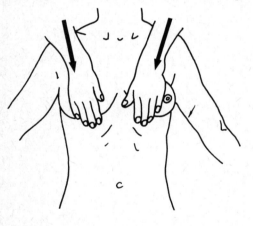

NOTE: For partner shiatsu, repeat shiatsu to the legs/feet and arms/hands for the right side.

ABDOMEN

As mentioned previously, it is best to begin a complete session with the neck and finish with the abdomen. These are the two most important areas and require the most care. When giving shiatsu to the abdomen, direct skin contact is preferable, and be sure your hands are warm. Do not give shiatsu to the abdomen when your partner's stomach is empty or too full. Wait about forty minutes after a meal. Your partner should use the toilet, if necessary, beforehand.

The aim is to release tension in the abdomen. Hardness or

pliancy should be carefully gauged in each area, and pressure adjusted so that the shiatsu remains pleasant for the receiver. Once you have become accustomed to the procedure, shiatsu to the abdominal region should last from five to ten minutes. Children must be treated very gently.

Shiatsu given regularly to this region will strengthen the stomach and liver, stimulate the intestines, and aid digestion. It is particularly helpful for children with indigestion or poor appetite (see Shiatsu for Children). Shiatsu to the solar plexus tones the diaphragm muscles and contributes greatly to the health of the abdominal organs.

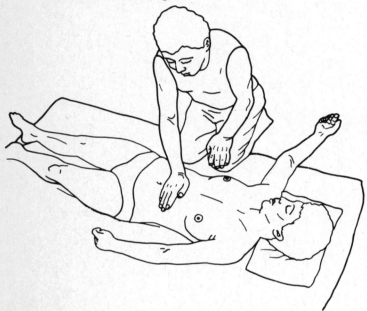

1. Have your partner lie on her back with legs extended and hands resting lightly on her chest, or with her right arm extended straight out and her left arm at her side. Kneel at your partner's right side, facing her abdomen.

Place your left hand on your left knee and, with your right palm, press lightly on the solar plexus (page 19). This point corresponds to the stomach. Notice whether this point is stretched tight like the skin of a drum or is soft and flabby. Neither extreme is good. Elasticity indicates good health. Next, notice the pulse at this point. It should be neither too strong nor too weak. A proper pulse also indicates good health. Now apply slightly stronger pressure and notice if there is any stiffness.

In this way, proceed to press the other nine points, which correspond to 2. small intestine, 3. bladder, 4. ascending colon, 5. liver, 6. stomach (repeated slightly lower), 7. spleen, 8. descending colon, 9. sigmoid colon (the S-shaped section just above the rectum), and 10. rectum. Repeat twice.

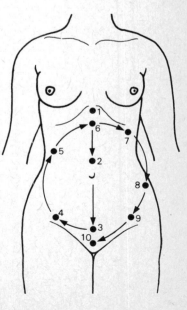

2. Apply palm pressure to the eight points of the small intestine surrounding the navel, starting from the topmost point and working clockwise. Repeat twice.

SELF-SHIATSU: First apply overlapping-palm pressure to the ten-point series in step 1, then to the eight points around the navel.

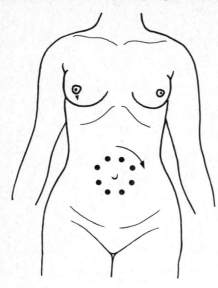

3. Place your left hand lightly on your partner's right hip for support and, with the fleshy part of your right palm near the base of the thumb, apply pressure to the four points shown using a kneading movement in a slightly downward direction. Repeat twice.

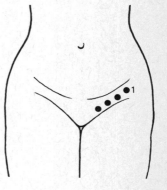

4. Kneel facing your partner's abdomen again. Place both palms on the stomach region so that the knuckles of the thumbs meet at the navel. Press with your fingers and pull toward you, then press with the heels of your hands and push away from you. Repeat this wavelike movement four times.

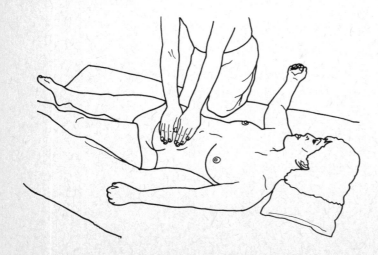

5. Raise your hips and, with both palms in the same position, apply deep pressure. Maintaining the pressure, move your palms in a clockwise circular motion ten times.

SELF-SHIATSU: Skip step 3 and follow the same procedures for steps 4 and 5, placing one hand over the other just above the navel. Finish with a vibrating pressure for ten seconds. The full-body self-shiatsu procedure ends here.

6. Shift your position and raise your hips and left knee so that you are looking down at the lower abdominal region. Place the heels of both palms on the hipbone where it protrudes on each side of the abdomen. Press the left side, then the right, one second each, alternating rhythmically ten times.

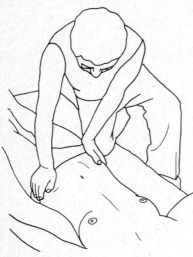

7. Have your partner place her hands above her head, with fingers curled. Slide both hands under the back directly below the navel until your fingertips meet. Bracing the backs of your hands on the floor, apply upward kneading pressure with your fingers on both sides of the spine. Only your fingers should move. Repeat twice. It is an indication of good health if this area is pliant and lifts easily.

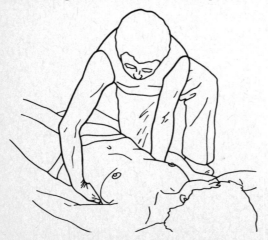

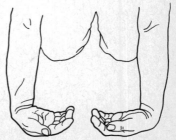

8. Remaining in the same position, place both hands on the sides of the abdomen, fingers pointing down. Press and then pull upward quickly, bringing the palms together above the navel. Repeat twice.

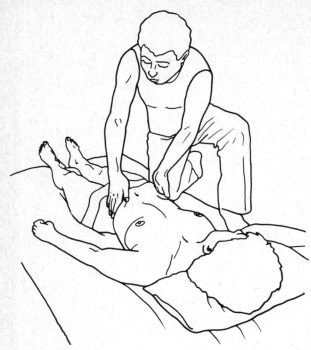

9. Stroke rapidly and smoothly down the abdomen from the solar plexus. Do ten times, alternating left and right palms.

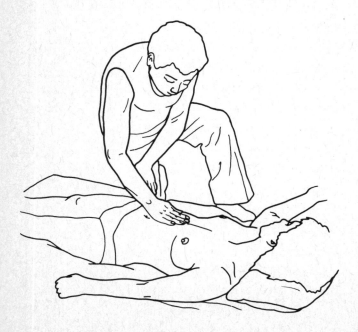

10. With overlapping palms (left over right at a ninety-degree angle), apply vibrating pressure over the navel for ten seconds.

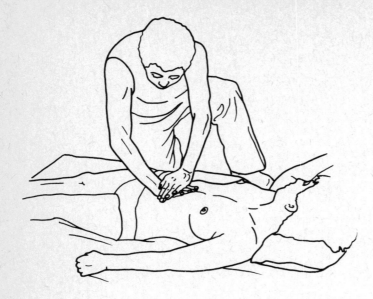

INCREASING VITALITY

Many of us are kept from leading a more vigorous, healthy, and fulfilling life by nagging physical complaints, which may have a great variety of causes. Whether the problems stem from emotional, dietary, environmental, or other causes, they may become, if neglected over the years, more severe and require lengthy and expensive medical treatment. This chapter will give you procedures to use on a regular basis to tone and stimulate the internal organs that are most prone to trouble. You will be giving preventive care, as well as improving the functioning of the body's systems. This chapter will also give shiatsu procedures for increasing sexual vitality.

STRENGTHENING THE HEART

Heart disease has become more and more widespread in modern society. Among the reasons are excessive cholesterol and sugar intake, lack of exercise, excess weight, and cigarette smoking. All these factors can lead to arteriosclerosis and its accompanying symptoms: palpitations, shortness of breath, and tightness in the chest. Although shiatsu is valuable as an early-stage preventive, you must also take steps to decrease your consumption of stimulants, watch your diet, and get regular exercise. Cardiac irregularities are often reflected as pain or stiffness in the body, particularly in the left side of the chest, the base and inside of the left arm, the left ring and little fingers, and the solar plexus.

1. Spread the fingers of your right hand and place them so that the index, middle, and ring fingers fit between the ribs on your left side. Apply pressure to the two sets of three horizontal rows between the ribs, working from the breastbone outward, and from top to bottom, three rows at a time.

2. Apply three-finger pressure with the right hand to the points along the groove where the arm meets the chest.

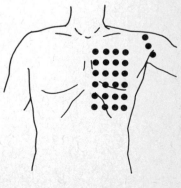

3. With your right thumb, apply pressure first to the pulse point in the armpit (to locate, see page 41, step 1). Press in the direction of the base of the neck. Repeat twice. Then continue along the five remaining points on the inside of the upper arm.

4. With your thumb, press the eight points along the lower inside edge of the lower arm from the elbow to the wrist.

5. Holding your left little finger between your right thumb and index finger, apply pressure to the points from the base to the tip of the finger, then pull. Repeat for your left ring finger.

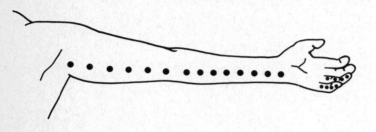

6. Place your left hand on your right shoulder, then reach under your left arm to your back with your right hand. Apply three-finger pressure to the points between the left shoulder blade and the spine, then to the points on the outer edge of the shoulder blade.

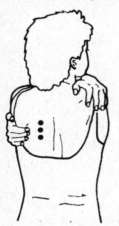

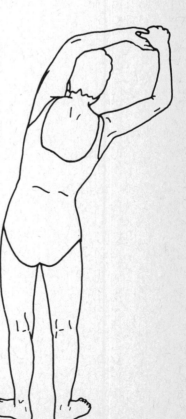

7. Grasp the base of your left little finger with your right hand and, leaning slightly to the right, stretch your left arm over your head for ten seconds. Repeat for your left ring finger and again with the little and ring fingers held together.

8. Apply three-finger pressure with your right hand to the upper-shoulder point (see first illustration). Finally, press your solar plexus (page 19) with overlapping palms. Repeat once.

STRENGTHENING THE LIVER

The liver is the largest of the digestive organs. Two-thirds of it lies under the protection of the right rib cage. In Japanese it is called the "silent giant," because, unlike the heart and stomach, it works quietly and unnoticeably. It performs numerous functions, among them detoxification and metabolism of fats, proteins, and carbohydrates; it also serves as a storehouse of energy. Overeating, excessive alcohol consumption, and fatigue can lead to liver disorders that progress to serious stages without manifesting any particularly noticeable symptoms.

The Japanese adage "Anger destroys the liver" is certainly true. Stress and emotional upset interfere with the proper functioning of the liver and are behind many liver problems. Irregularities of the liver appear as stiffness and pain in the right shoulder, between the lower right shoulder blade and the spine, and at the lower edge of the right rib cage from the solar plexus to the right upper abdomen.

1. Apply overlapping-palm pressure (left over right) to the four points along the lower edge of the right rib cage, working from top to bottom. Repeat once.

2. Apply three-finger pressure with the left hand to the right upper-shoulder point.

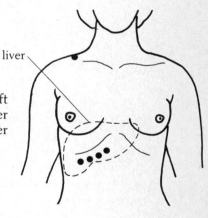

liver

3. Place your right hand on your left shoulder; then, with your left hand, reach around beneath your right arm and apply three-finger pressure to the points between the spine and the lower shoulder blade. You may need help with these points.

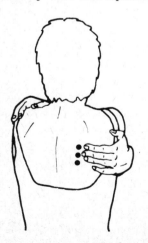

4. With overlapping palms, press as though pulling down on the liver and hold for five seconds. Repeat three times.

STRENGTHENING THE ABDOMINAL ORGANS

When muscular tension builds up in the abdomen, it is easy to become angry or upset, and the abdominal organs are easily damaged. Keeping the abdominal organs relaxed makes it easier to respond to people and events more calmly. If you make the time to give yourself shiatsu for the abdomen every day for five minutes, the proper functioning of your abdominal organs will be restored, your digestion will be efficient, your stamina will increase, and the muscles throughout your body will become more flexible.

When applying shiatsu to the abdominal region, the first aim is to release the tension in the solar plexus (points 1 and 6). These points are connected reflexively to all the abdominal organs.

1. Place overlapping palms (left on right) over the solar plexus and inhale, then exhale slowly as you press for three seconds. Do five times.

2. Using the same pressure, press the ten abdominal points in order. Repeat three times.

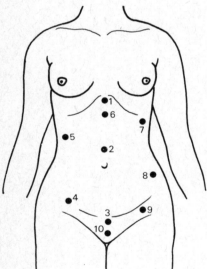

3. Apply overlapping palms to the eight points around the navel. Repeat twice.

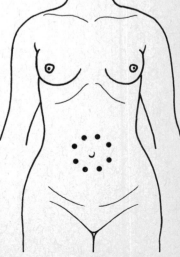

4. Apply the same pressure to the points running diagonally to the lower left of the navel. Repeat twice.

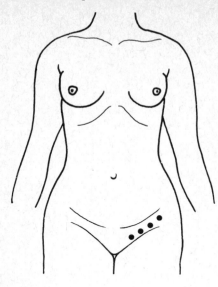

5. Place both hands, palms overlapping, firmly over the navel and apply suction pressure with a clockwise circular movement ten times. Then apply soft vibration for ten seconds.

KIDNEY AILMENTS

Acute kidney ailments accompanied by fever require prompt diagnosis and medical treatment. However, if you are troubled by weak kidneys, you may suffer from such symptoms as fatigue, headache, dizziness, and swelling. You may have a greater volume of urine at night than during the day and find yourself getting up again and again to urinate. These are signs of a chronic kidney ailment.

kidneys

bladder

1. The kidneys are located on either side of the backbone about even with the navel. First, give thorough shiatsu to the ten back points using slow, gentle pressure over the kidneys (the third through fifth points).

2. Link your hands behind your back and press the kidneys with the heels of your hands.

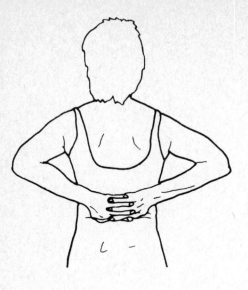

3. The kidneys respond well to shiatsu to the arches of the feet. Give special attention to the three points on the inside of the arch with strong thumb pressure.

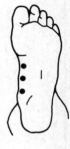

4. Stimulating the abdominal organs will also help the kidneys. Apply overlapping-palm pressure with both hands to the ten abdominal points. Then apply deep palm pressure on either side of the navel.

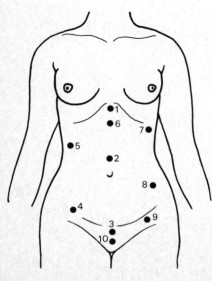

INCREASING SEXUAL VITALITY

Just as your digestive system functions best when you eat in a calm, relaxed atmosphere, your enjoyment of sex is maximized when you are fully relaxed and free from strain. In the life of any couple, there are bound to be times of physical or mental trouble. These are the times a couple most needs mutual help and encouragement, as well as strength and good health. Giving each other shiatsu is a wonderful way for a couple to develop the ability to deal with difficulties and to maintain vigorous good health.

For whatever reason, when the muscles throughout the body are tense and inflexible, sexual sensitivity is dulled. It is particularly important to maintain flexibility and muscle tone in the lower back and legs by getting adequate exercise. It is said that aging begins with the legs; as the legs become weaker, sexual feeling also weakens. Shiatsu can help to tone muscles. Also, remember to give regular shiatsu to the medulla oblongata, the front of the neck (for the thyroid gland), and the adrenal glands (located at the top of the kidneys) to maintain proper hormone secretion.

Impotence and frigidity also lead to deteriorating sexual relations. Shiatsu works both directly and indirectly to relieve or ease psychological and physical factors. Impotence may be caused by physical or mental fatigue or by poor nutrition. Psychological factors, such as feelings of physical inferiority, may also be involved. In men past middle age, sexual vigor declines with physical vigor, but in recent years impotence has been increasing in younger men. Such cases are not usually caused by physical abnormality, but by psychological problems, stress, or mental exhaustion.

Frigidity, except for cases when there are physical abnormalities in the sexual organs, nearly always stems from mental causes. However, that does not mean the problem is always in the woman's mind. Often male insensitivity, ignorance, or premature ejaculation are factors in female frigidity. Sex in which both partners do not receive pleasure is empty and meaningless.

With regular practice each partner will develop the sensitivity to recognize and respond to the other's weak points and areas of stress. In addition to toning and stimulating key areas of the body, practicing shiatsu as a couple can help to create the relaxed and caring atmosphere that is conducive to sexual satisfaction. (See also Preventing Prostrate Trouble.)

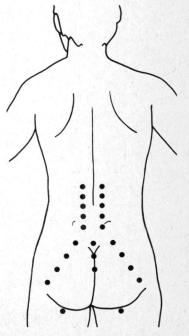

1. Have your partner lie on her stomach. First press the five lower-back points with overlapping thumbs, giving strong pressure to the fifth point.

2. Next, apply two-thumb pressure to the three rows of points on the buttocks. Use overlapping-thumb pressure for the Namikoshi points (page 18).

3. Apply gradually increasing, upward pressure to the lowest point of the middle row at the base of the tailbone.

4. Apply upward kneading pressure to the two points on the buttocks where the buttocks meet the legs.

5. Reach beneath the hips with both hands to the points just to the inside of the hipbone and apply three-finger pressure with a slow, upward kneading motion, alternating from right to left.

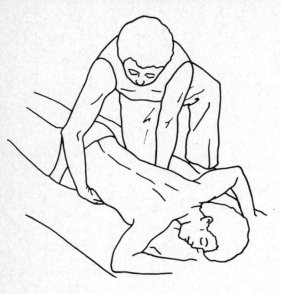

6. Press the base of each toe, top and bottom simultaneously; then, while pulling gently, shake the toe to "vibrate" it. Press the arch point of each foot with overlapping thumbs.

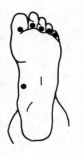

7. Have your partner turn over. Apply palm pressure to the lower abdominal points, numbers 3 and 10. Give particular attention to the last point over the pubic bone.

8. Apply palm pressure to the two rows of groin points.

9. Press the first five points on the inner thighs with overlapping thumbs.

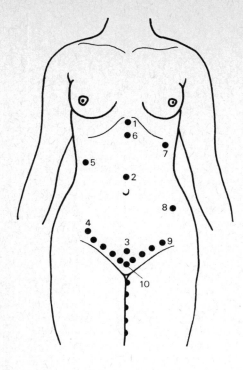

10. For women, hold the breasts between thumbs and fingers, and press firmly at the base. Then hold the nipples between thumb and forefinger and pull gently. For men, cup the fingers around the scrotum and with the thumbs, press gently at the base of the penis.

RELIEVING STRESS AND FATIGUE

Fatigue may be a result of physical exhaustion or mental strain. Regardless of cause, fatigue will sap your energy and sooner or later take a toll on your health. It is probably fair to say that most people in today's stressful urban environments suffer from too much tension. Both fatigue and stress impede the natural functioning of the body's systems.

This chapter will emphasize ways to use shiatsu to cope with fatigue and stress in your daily life. When you become aware of tiredness or discomfort, take a few minutes to give shiatsu to the affected area. You will not only feel more energized, alert, and relaxed, but you will be preventing the development of more serious health problems. By learning to care for yourself and others in this way, you will develop an attitude that itself will contribute to your well-being and enjoyment of life.

These procedures are given primarily for self-shiatsu, but you may easily adapt them for partner shiatsu by using the appropriate sections of full-body shiatsu. When instructions are given for the left side, be sure to give shiatsu to the right side, too—or instead, when appropriate. Most procedures may be repeated according to individual needs.

MENTAL FATIGUE

The brain requires adequate stimulation and a continuous supply of fresh blood for proper functioning. When blood flow to the brain is sluggish or irregular, memory is dulled, the head feels heavy, and headaches and insomnia occur.

1. Apply overlapping three-finger pressure to the points along the median line from the hairline to the crown of the head.

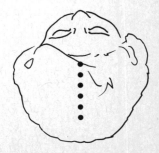

2. Apply three-finger pressure with the left and right hands simultaneously to the six rows of three points each on either side of the median line. Start from the crown of the head and finish at the hairline, working outward from the median line.

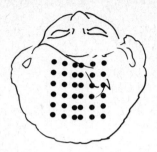

3. Apply pressure with overlapping palms to the front, crown, and back of the head, then with both palms simultaneously to the sides of the head.

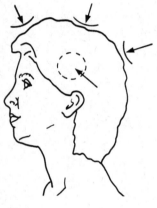

EYESTRAIN

When you are suffering from eyestrain and its accompanying symptoms—eye pain, blurred vision, and headaches—you probably think in terms of strain from excessive typing, reading, driving, and so forth. However, lack of sleep, stiff shoulders or neck, air pollution, or a lack of vitamin A may also be contributing factors. Shiatsu releases tension in the muscles around your eyes and may even improve vision, but you should also make an effort to rest your eyes at regular intervals, particularly when doing eye-fatiguing work.

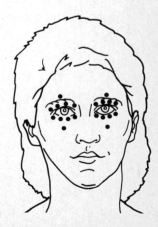

1. Apply three-finger pressure with both hands simultaneously to the points along each upper eye socket, working outward, then to the points along each lower eye socket.

2. Use three-finger pressure on the point at the center of each cheekbone. Next, with overlapping fingers (middle over index), press the point over the center of each eyebrow.

3. Apply three-finger pressure with both hands simultaneously to each horizontal row, beginning each time with the points closest to the eyes. Do the center rows first, followed by top and bottom.

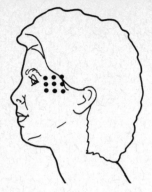

4. Using three-finger pressure, place the fingers beneath the eyes and move them slowly across the points of the eye sockets, pulling the skin outward as you go. Hold the position at the last point for ten seconds. Do the same above the eyes. Repeat twice.

5. Repeat this pulling pressure for the temple points.

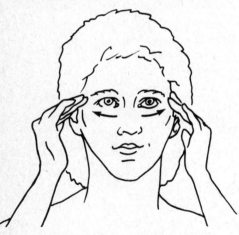

6. Rotate your eyes ten times to the left, then ten times to the right.

7. Place the palms of the hands over the eyes and press the eye sockets lightly for ten seconds.

STIFF SHOULDER

Muscle fatigue from heavy work or tension often leads to stiffness in the shoulder area. In addition, abnormalities in the heart or stomach are reflected on the surface of the body as stiffness in the left shoulder, and in the liver or gallbladder as stiffness in the right shoulder. By applying pressure to the shoulder area, the reflexive connection between the surface of the body and the internal organs is stimulated, and normal functioning is restored.

1. With your right hand, apply three-finger pressure to the point on your left upper shoulder at the base of the neck. Press for five seconds in the direction of a point level with the solar plexus along the central axis of the body.

2. From this point, press the points along the upper shoulder muscle, then the three points along the muscle that connects to the shoulder blade. Repeat steps 1 and 2 three to five times, depending on the degree of stiffness. Repeat for your right shoulder.

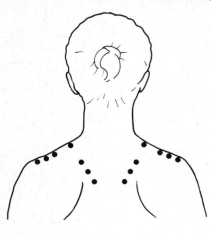

3. Lift your shoulders up in a slow shrugging motion, then let them drop. Do five times. Lift your shoulders, shift them forward, and let them drop. Lift again, shift them back, and drop them once more. Do five times.

LOWER BACK PAIN

The main cause of lower back pain is irregularity in the natural curvature of the lower spine from sitting or standing in the same position for a long time. Lower back pain will occur if the curvature of the spine becomes greater than normal and the abdomen protrudes, or if it becomes less than normal and the lower back loses its natural curve.

1. Use your thumbs to apply pressure simultaneously to the five points on each side of the lower spine, then to the three points on each side along the upper edge of the hipbone.

2. Lie on your right side and, with your left thumb, press the five points on the left side of your lower spine. Reverse your position and repeat for your right side.

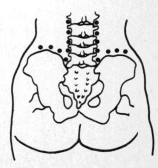

For too much curvature:

1. Lie on your back, raise your head and torso, wrap your arms around your legs, and pull your knees as close to your face as you can. Hold this position for ten seconds, then lower your head and legs and relax. Repeat twice.

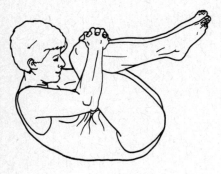

2. Stand facing a wall at arm's length. Place your palms firmly against the wall at about shoulder level. Pull in your abdomen and straighten your back for ten seconds. Repeat twice.

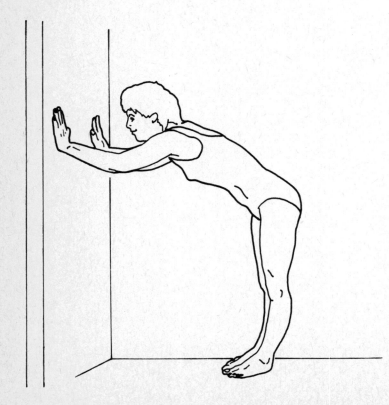

For too little curvature:

1. Lie facedown, bend your knees, raise your torso off the floor as much as you can, grasp your feet or ankles with both hands, and stretch for ten seconds. Repeat twice.

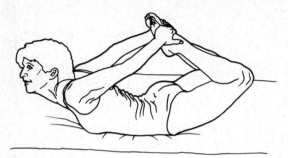

2. Stand with your back to a wall. Bend back as far as you can, brace yourself against the wall with your hands, and hold for ten seconds. Repeat twice.

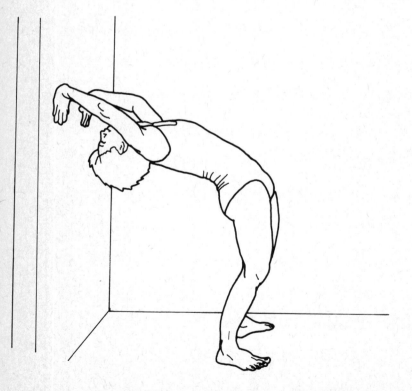

HEADACHE

Headaches have many causes, among them lack of sleep, hardening of the arteries, high blood pressure, constipation, premenstrual tension, stress, and fatigue. When you have a good idea of what the cause of your headache is, in addition to giving special attention to your head, you can give shiatsu to other areas of the body according to your specific circumstances. Often when you do not know what is causing your headache, there may be tension in your neck, shoulders, or back, which you have not even noticed. Be sure to give shiatsu to these areas too. Moreover, shiatsu to areas where the blood flow is sluggish stimulates circulation and helps to make you alert and clear-headed again.

A headache is nearly always accompanied by stiffness of the neck at the base of the skull. Apply shiatsu here first, before going on to the head.

1. Use three-finger pressure for all of the following steps. Follow steps 1 and 2 for Mental Fatigue (page 64).

2. Again press the points on each side of the median line, this time both sides at once. Repeat five times. Then press the six median points again, stopping at the last point on the crown. Increase the pressure gradually for five seconds, then release gently.

3. Press the three points along the median line of the forehead, working upward. Repeat twice.

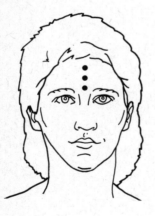

4. Press the three points along the median line of the back of the head, again three times. Apply deep pressure for five seconds to each of the three points at the base of the skull.

5. Finally, press the temples with the heels of your hands for five seconds.

MIGRAINE

Migraine headaches are characterized by severe pain noticeably stronger on one side of the head. The pain may be localized, running from the front of the head to the eyes, or concentrated in the temples. Although their cause is not well understood, it is known that tension in the shoulder and neck muscles may trigger migraines. Shiatsu to the abdominal area is also helpful in cases of migraine. Blood circulation in the abdominal organs is stimulated, which in turn helps to relieve the headache.

1. First apply shiatsu to the neck muscles on the side that the migraine is concentrated on. Press the three rows of points, with three-finger pressure from top to bottom, beginning with the front row (page 22).

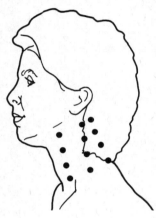

2. Pay special attention to the medulla oblongata (page 18). Use overlapping middle fingers.

3. Apply three-finger pressure to the upper-shoulder points.

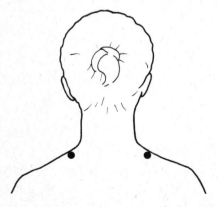

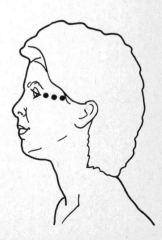

4. Follow step 2 for Headaches (on facing page).

5. Apply three-finger pressure to the three temple points.

6. Apply palm pressure to the side of the head in which the migraine is concentrated, supporting the other side of the head with your other hand.

HANGOVER

Excessive drinking typically leads to a hangover, which makes itself felt in the form of nausea, dizziness, and severe headache. These symptoms are caused by residual alcohol in the body, which excites the nervous system, stimulates abnormal secretion of stomach acids, and causes abnormal fermentation in the digestive tract. Since heavy drinking places an extra burden on the stomach as well as the liver, the last two steps in this sequence are especially important.

1. Place your left thumb gently on the pulse point beneath the jaw on the left side of the front of the neck. This is a vital point on the carotid artery, which regulates blood flow to the head, and the vagus nerve, which leads to the internal organs. Press the points from this point to the collarbone for two to three seconds each. Repeat twice, then press the right side.

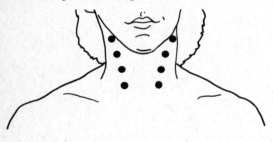

2. Apply palm pressure to the sides of the head for ten seconds.

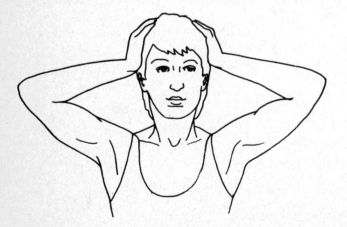

3. Apply strong pressure to the medulla oblongata (page 18) with overlapping middle fingers for five seconds. Repeat twice.

4. Apply overlapping-palm pressure to the solar plexus (see page 20) for three seconds. Do ten times.

5. Apply overlapping palms to the liver point, just below the rib cage on the right side, again for three seconds. Do ten times.

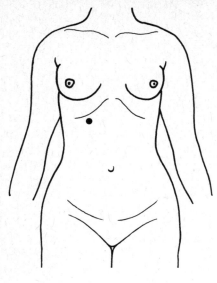

STOMACHACHE

In Japan, the stomach or abdomen is considered the seat of the emotions. Indeed, its condition is closely tied to one's emotional state. In times of prolonged anxiety and stress, the secretion of gastric juices increases, and their acidity irritates the mucous membrane lining of the stomach, causing stomach distress. The reason you lose your appetite when you have a sudden emotional upset is, again, the abnormal secretion of gastric juices. A persistent state of distress will cause nervous indigestion, and when further aggravated may lead to gastric ulcers. People who are temperamentally inclined to such stomach problems must make a regular effort to relieve the strain and anxiety which lead to stomach irritation.

Before the onset of a stomachache there is sure to be stiffness in the muscles of the neck and shoulders, especially the left shoulder and between the left shoulder blade and the spine. It is essential to give shiatsu to these areas regularly to relax tension. When a stomachache has already started, rather than suddenly pushing on the upper abdomen, work on relaxing these muscles first.

1. First, lie on your back and apply overlapping-palm pressure to the solar plexus (page 19), exhaling and relaxing as you press. The solar plexus is likely to be tight at first, so press lightly and gradually increase until you can press deeply. You may find that lying with your knees bent helps you relax at first.

2. You will need a partner's help for the points between your shoulder blades. Lie on your right side with your left knee bent. Have your partner apply overlapping-thumb pressure to the lower three points between the left shoulder blade and the spine. Then lie facedown and have your partner apply thumb pressure to the same points, right and left sides simultaneously.

ACID INDIGESTION

The gastric juices secreted in the stomach aid in digestion and kill bacteria. But they contain acid which, when secreted in abnormal quantities, irritates the stomach lining and causes belching and a bitter taste in tne mouth. Frequent acid indigestion can lead to gastric ulcers, so if you are prone to this problem, you must be careful not to abuse your stomach. Eat a balanced diet, low in meats and starches; do not overeat; and avoid alcohol, tobacco, and coffee. Also, try to reduce stress and nervous excitement in your daily life.

1. First, apply thumb pressure to the top points on the front of the neck (left side, then right; page 22). Repeat twice. This will stimulate the autonomic nerves and normalize the secretion of gastric juices.

2. Apply overlapping-palm pressure to the solar plexus (points 1 and 6) for five seconds. Do ten times.

3. Apply overlapping-palm pressure to all ten abdominal points to stimulate the digestive organs.

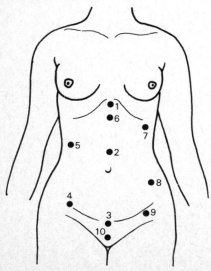

4. Press the shoulders at the base of the neck, then press all the back points (the five upper back points and the ten lower), giving particular attention to the third, fourth, and fifth points between the left shoulder blade and the spine. You will need a partner's help for these points.

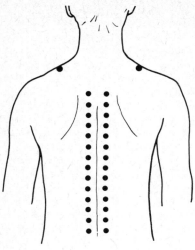

HEARTBURN

Heartburn is characterized by a burning sensation from the area of the solar plexus and an unpleasant feeling of constriction in the chest. It may also be accompanied by nausea and belching. It is usually brought on by eating too fast or too much, or from eating too much heavy, starchy food. Anyone may get heartburn once in a while, but if it occurs frequently, it may indicate the early stages of a more serious stomach disorder.

1. Apply three-finger pressure to the upper-shoulder points.

2. Apply thumb pressure to both sides of the upper back. You will need a partner's help here.

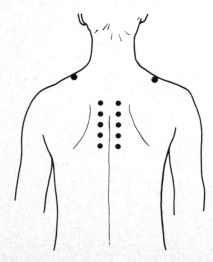

3. Press the abdominal points with overlapping palms. Repeat once. Give particular attention to the solar plexus (points 1 and 6).

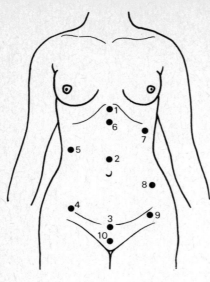

4. With fingers spread, press the rows between the ribs (a finger to each row, three rows at a time). Do both sides at the same time.

5. Gently press the five breastbone points using three-finger pressure with both hands.

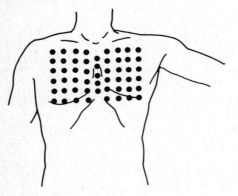

6. For men, apply circular palm pressure to the chest ten times, then stroke downward and inward to the solar plexus ten times. For women, stroke downward from the upper chest to the beginning of the breasts.

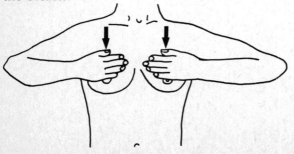

DROWSINESS

Everyone knows the terrible feeling of wanting to close his eyes and doze off when he must stay awake: at meetings, lectures—a list of such occasions would be endless. But the one that is particularly dangerous is dozing at the wheel. When you feel drowsy while driving, stop and give yourself a moment of shiatsu, maybe even as you wait at a stoplight.

1. Apply fairly strong pressure for three seconds to the two points on the inner upper edge of each eye socket, being careful not to press on the eyeball. Apply pressure with overlapping middle and index fingers. Repeat twice.

2. Apply three-finger pressure to the eight points around the eye sockets. Repeat twice.

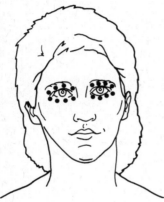

3. Press the three temple points with three-finger pressure. Apply fairly strong pressure to the first point. Repeat twice.

4. Apply strong three-finger pressure for three seconds to the point behind the earlobe and just below the small projecting part of the skull behind the ear. Repeat twice.

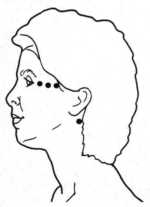

5. Apply strong pressure for five seconds to the medulla oblongata (page 18) with overlapping middle fingers. Repeat twice.

6. Place both palms over the eyes for ten seconds, then remove them quickly.

INSOMNIA

People who suffer from insomnia tend to be subject to nervousness and anxiety. They are easily worried, irritated, or angered. They become upset when they can't sleep, making it even more difficult to fall asleep, and in desperation often resort to sleeping pills. Insomniacs may fall into this vicious circle; typically tension has built up in the neck, shoulder, and abdominal areas as a result. As you learn to release the tension in these areas, you should gradually be able to resume your normal sleeping patterns.

1. Begin at the pulse point of the carotid artery, which is the uppermost point on the left front of the neck. (This important shiatsu point regulates the heart, blood pressure, and blood supply to the brain. Do not press too long or strongly on this point.) From here, press the remaining three neck points for two to three seconds each. Repeat twice, then do the right side.

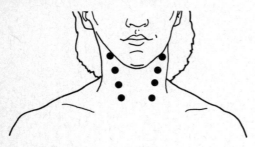

2. Use three-finger pressure to press the row on each side of the neck simultaneously. Repeat twice.

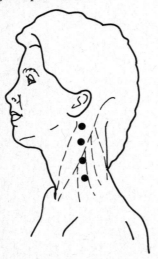

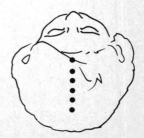

3. Apply three-finger pressure with both hands to the points along the median line of the head from the hairline to the crown. Repeat twice. Press the last point three more times.

4. Press the points along the median line of the back of the head three times. Press the medulla oblongata (page 18) for five seconds with overlapping middle fingers. Repeat twice.

5. Use three-finger pressure on the upper shoulder points—left, then right. Repeat twice.

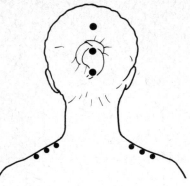

6. Apply palm pressure to the ten abdominal points in order. Repeat two to four times.

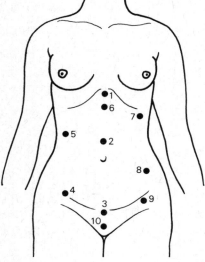

DIFFICULTY IN WAKING

Rising from bed in the morning can be a trying experience when you must fight a lethargic body or clouded head. The fatigue from the previous day is still with you. This is because the brain is tired from overuse and sluggish with stale blood full of toxins. This heavy-headed, exhausted feeling will not go away until the brain is supplied with fresh blood. The brain will remain in a kind of overexcited state. People who do intellectual labor are prone to this trouble. Shiatsu to the head and carotid artery will stimulate blood flow to the brain.

Many people complain of a stiff neck in the morning. The muscles are so tight, the neck can hardly turn. It only takes a few moments of shiatsu to relieve these heavy, unpleasant feel-ings and help you function more effectively. You can do it anywhere, alone or with friends. It is also quite beneficial when you have been doing desk work for two or three hours and are starting to feel groggy.

1. Follow steps 1 and 2 for Mental Fatigue (page 66).

2. Apply three-finger pressure to the back of the head with both hands simultaneously.

3. Link your fingers behind your head and press the neck point with your thumbs.

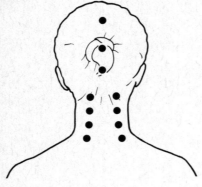

4. Press the points down the center of the forehead, then the temples.

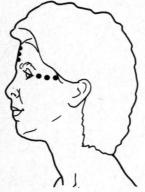

5. Apply thumb pressure to the points on the front of the neck, first left, then right. Press gently and repeatedly. The blood vessels will expand and your head will feel much lighter.

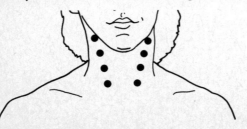

KNEE PAIN

When the legs are not used enough, the muscles, tendons, and cartilage of the knees become stiff and the knee joints lose flexibility. Then, when the joints are subjected to unusual use, the cartilage wears away, altering the structure of the joints and resulting in restricted movement, pain, swelling, and water on the knees. When the natural spaces in the joints become constricted, the knees make the grating, snapping noises familiar to so many people. Excess weight in this condition puts an even greater burden on already vulnerable knees.

1. Apply two-thumb pressure to the points surrounding the kneecap, five above and five below.

2. Apply two-thumb pressure to the points along the muscle above and below the knee, working downward.

3. Place your palm firmly over the kneecap and rotate your hand gently clockwise ten times, then counterclockwise ten times. Then vibrate your hand for ten seconds. Repeat once.

4. Apply three-finger pressure with both hands to each of the three vertical rows on the back of the knee.

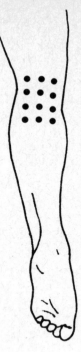

Exercises

1. Stand on your right foot and tuck your left leg under, holding your left ankle in your left hand. Pull it as close to your left buttock as you can and hold for ten seconds. Repeat twice.

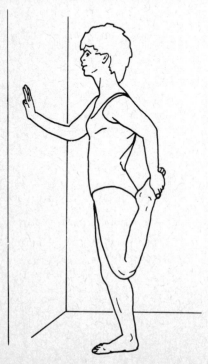

2. Stand and bend your knees slightly. Place your hands on your knees and, without moving your feet, rotate your knees ten times in a wide circle, then rotate ten times in the other direction.

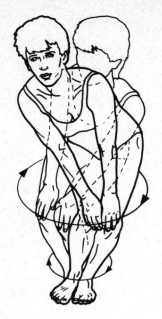

TIRED ARMS

Stiff shoulders and backache are common enough problems, but sometimes the arms too become stiff and sore, especially from housework, unaccustomed weekend exercise, or sports like tennis or golf. If you start the workweek with this kind of fatigue, on Friday you may find yourself wondering why you have so little energy. Only a few minutes of shiatsu can be quite invigorating.

Press all the arm points, following the procedure given on pages 41–44.

TIRED FEET AND CALVES

1. Holding your left foot by the ankle, press the points (front and back) on the toes with your thumb and index finger three times.

2. Apply thumb pressure to the four rows of points between the bones running from the base of the toes to the base of the ankle. Repeat once or twice. Press the three points across the front of the ankle.

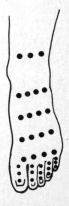

3. Press the inner and outer sides of the heel, slowly and thoroughly.

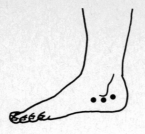

4. Press the arch of the foot. The arch points are very important for relieving fatigue because they are the reflex points for the kidneys. (You can gauge how tired you are by the degree of tenderness you feel when you press here. Shiatsu applied to the arch not only relieves fatigue but helps prevent kidney disorders.)

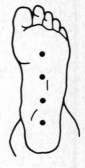

5. Press the first lateral shin point (page 19) strongly with overlapping thumbs. This is the point to press when your knees feel like jelly from overexertion.

6. Press the six points from the first lateral shin point to the ankle.

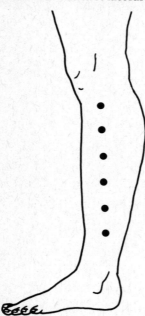

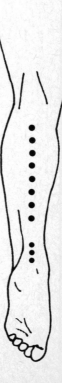

7. Press the eight points along the calf muscle and the three along the Achilles tendon.

TREATING
COMMON
DISORDERS

Shiatsu can be beneficial in treating many common disorders. It should not be used as a substitute for professional medical care. However, it may be used to cure minor conditions and to aid healing in many circumstances. These procedures are for common temporary disorders that can be easily treated at home.

ANKLE SPRAIN

Ankle sprains often occur when you are fatigued, momentarily lose your balance, or slip going downhill or down a set of stairs. A sprain means that the tendons and ligaments that protect the ankle are stretched and blood vessels are torn, causing internal bleeding accompanied by painful swelling and inflammation. When this happens, wrap the ankle immediately in a bandage and do not put any weight on the foot. (Or, in an emergency, apply a temporary bandage over the shoe and pant leg to support the ankle.)

If there is swelling or inflammation, apply a cold, damp cloth and keep the ankle still. Do not begin shiatsu treatment until the pain and swelling have gone down.

Shiatsu treatment can speed recovery from a sprain and prevent aftereffects. If the ligaments remain stiff and extended after a sprain, the ankle will be weakened and may become painful with changes in weather, but conscientious shiatsu treatment can help facilitate full recovery.

1. Press the points around the ankle, three on the outside and three on the inside. *For all steps, press very gently at first.*

2. Apply thumb pressure to the points on the instep.

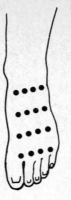

3. Finish with thumb pressure to the arch and heel.

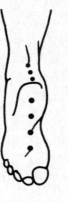

4. Gently rotate the ankle, then bend the foot forward and back.

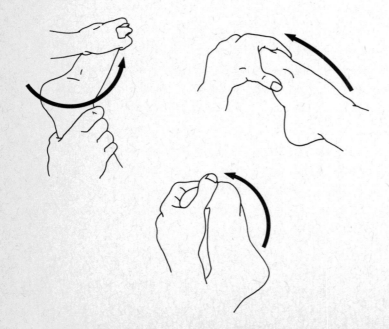

PULLED MUSCLE

When the body is extremely tired, the muscles lose their elasticity. Strain may become concentrated and a sudden movement is likely to result in a pulled muscle. Pulls are apt to occur just when you move to turn over in bed, unconsciously putting sudden and additional strain on the muscles. Most people are particularly susceptible to pulls in the summer when they perspire and lie uncovered in the chilly breeze of an air conditioner or fan. Pulled muscles occur in the neck, at the base of the shoulders, in the back (particularly between the shoulder blades), and in the chest between the ribs.

When treating a pull with shiatsu, do not apply strong, sudden pressure to the pulled muscle itself, but use gentle palm pressure to relax the general area, then use thumb or three-finger pressure to work gradually deeper into the center of the muscle. Move the muscle as little as possible until it is restored to its normal state. If possible, give shiatsu in a hot bath and be careful to avoid chilling afterward. Once a muscle has been pulled, reoccurrence is likely, so continue shiatsu to the area for several days.

CRAMPS OF THE CALF MUSCLE

Cramping in the calf muscle can be extremely painful because the muscle spasm often exerts pressure on a nerve. It is likely to occur when the calf muscles are fatigued, when you are not drinking enough fluids, or when you have diarrhea. In general, dehydration encourages cramps. They commonly happen at night because the muscles are apt to become chilled and stiff.

Cramps may also be caused by congestion of the veins of the legs due to poor circulation, pain in the hips, or chilling. They can become an ongoing problem, so regular shiatsu to keep the muscles pliant is a good preventive measure.

1. Apply palm pressure to the ten abdominal points.

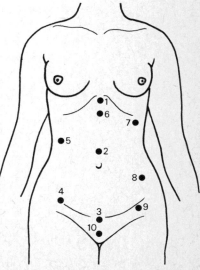

2. Press the eight points around the navel with the palm.

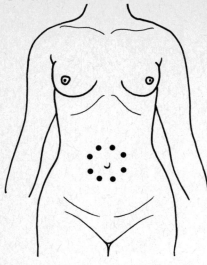

3. Press the ten lower-back points. Apply strong thumb pressure to the Namikoshi points (page 18).

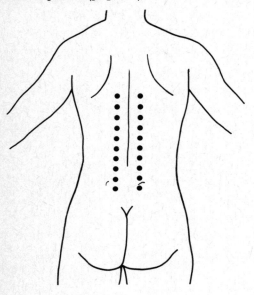

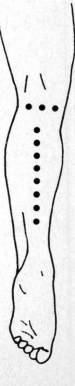

4. Apply three-finger pressure with both hands to the points on the back of the knee. Repeat twice.

5. Apply three-finger pressure with both hands to the eight points on the back of the calf.

6. Grasp the toes of the left foot with your right hand and pull back while applying thumb pressure with your left hand to the points along the outside of the shinbone. Repeat this procedure for the right leg.

7. Apply strong overlapping-thumb pressure to the uppermost point on the outside of the leg (the first lateral shin point; see also page 19) three times.

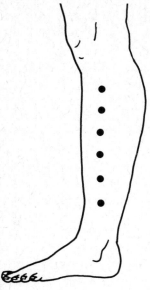

8. Use two-thumb pressure on the points on the sole of the foot, then apply strong pressure with overlapping thumbs to the third point from the top three times.

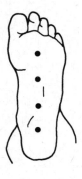

STOMACH CRAMP

Sudden sharp pains in the stomach are usually caused by spasms of the stomach muscles, although sharp pains on the right side may be due to gallstones. Causes are numerous, but nervous upset, which can strike anyone, is among the most common. The fifth upper-back point of the left side has long been known to be highly effective for relieving stomach cramps. You will need a partner's help for this treatment.

1. Lie on your stomach. Have your partner straddle you and then kneel, and apply strong pressure to the topmost back point on the left side with overlapping thumbs (left over right) for five seconds. (This is also the fifth upper-back point; see page 24). Repeat five or six times. This alone should bring relief.

2. If the cramps continue, have your partner press the ten points from this point down to the hips for three seconds each. After completing the left side, do the right. Repeat five or six times.

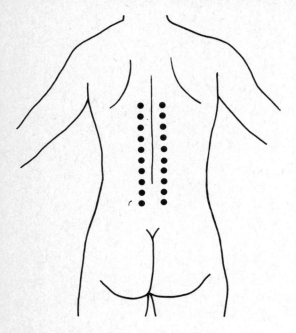

3. Turn over. Have your partner give light palm pressure to the solar plexus (page 19). Continued off and on for about five minutes, this should be very relaxing. You should rest quietly for a while afterward.

DIARRHEA

When the intestines are in poor condition, food is not digested completely. Excess gas and fermentation caused by digestive acids irritate the intestinal lining, causing increased peristaltic action and the watery stools of diarrhea. If this condition persists, absorption of nutrients stops and dehydration, loss of appetite, and lowered resistance to infection follow.

To restore proper functioning of the intestines, it is essential to give the digestive tract a chance to heal by eating mild foods in moderate quantities. If the condition persists for an abnormally long time, seek professional medical help. In times of fatigue, when the muscles become stiff, give preventive shiatsu to the abdomen to keep the digestive organs relaxed and functioning properly.

1. Apply strong pressure to the medulla oblongata (page 18) with overlapping middle fingers for five seconds. Do about five times.

2. Apply three-finger pressure to the upper-shoulder points for three seconds each. Do five times.

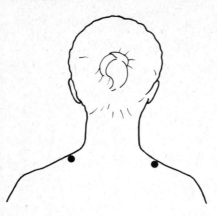

3. Apply strong thumb pressure simultaneously to both Namikoshi points (page 18) for five seconds. Do five to ten times.

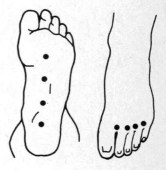

4. Apply overlapping-thumb pressure to the four points on the sole of the foot (giving especially strong pressure to the third), then to the four points on the top of the foot at the base of the toes, giving especially strong pressure to the first. Repeat twice.

5. Apply overlapping-palm pressure to the ten abdominal points.

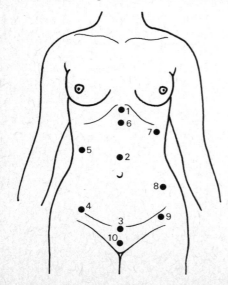

6. Use palm pressure again on the eight points around the navel. Repeat steps 5 and 6 two to four times.

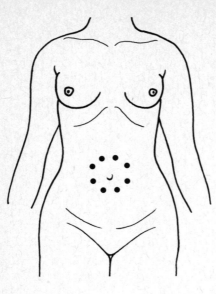

7. Apply palm pressure to both sides of the body in the area between the rib cage and the hipbones.

CONSTIPATION

Constipation may be caused by mental stress, changes in diet, or lack of exercise. Should irregular habits and poor digestion continue, the quantity of stool decreases, abdominal pressure decreases, and the movement of the intestines is weakened and chronic constipation may result.

Chronic constipation cannot be cured overnight by self-shiatsu, but with determination, patience, and daily application, great improvement can be achieved. Make it a habit to give yourself shiatsu in the morning before going to the toilet. It is helpful to have a cup of saltwater, Japanese green tea with a pickled plum (*umeboshi*), some fruit, or milk. The organic acid will stimulate the intestines.

Repeat the following procedure according to the severity of symptoms, but remember that the key to relief of chronic constipation is daily shiatsu.

1. First, apply thumb pressure to the points on each side of the front of the neck, one side at a time.

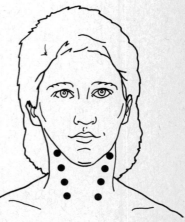

2. Press the medulla oblongata (page 18) with overlapping middle fingers.

3. Apply three-finger pressure to the upper-shoulder points, then the five lower-back points on either side of the spine.

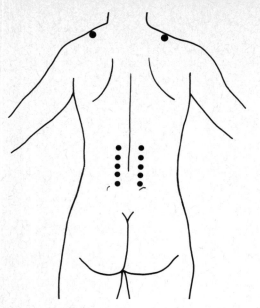

4. Apply strong thumb pressure simultaneously to both Namikoshi points (page 18).

5. Press the ten abdominal points—especially points seven, eight, nine, and ten—with overlapping palms.

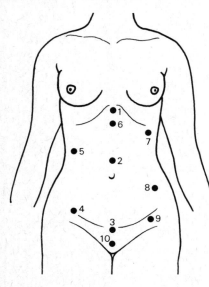

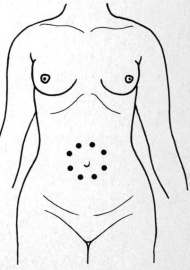

6. Use overlapping palms again to press the eight points around the navel.

BURSITIS

The shoulder joint has the greatest range of movement of any joint in the body and is surrounded by a complex arrangement of muscles and ligaments. Many people, when they reach late middle age, experience restricted movement in the shoulders. In Japan, this condition is called "fifties' shoulders." The shoulder muscles become so stiff, it is painful to lift the arms or rotate them backward. When the shoulders become fatigued, the muscles lose their flexibility, thus putting an extra burden on the tendons and making them prone to inflammation. Normal movement is impaired and pressure on the nerves causes pain.

1. Follow the first two steps for Stiff Shoulders (page 68).

2. Apply three-finger pressure to the three points down the center of the rounded part of the shoulder, then use opposing thumb and fingers to press the points on both sides.

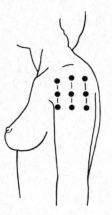

3. Place your left hand on your right shoulder and reach around with your right hand to your left shoulder blade and the base of the arm. Apply three-finger pressure to each of the three rows of three points, working from top to bottom and from the shoulder blade to the arm.

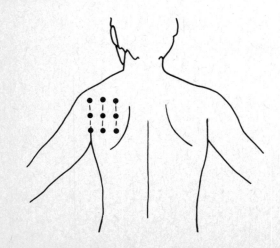

1. Hold a towel as you would when drying your back after a bath, with one hand up and the other down, and pull the towel back and forth. Reverse your hands and repeat.

2. With one elbow up and the other down, stretch gently to touch or clasp your fingertips behind your back. Reverse and repeat.

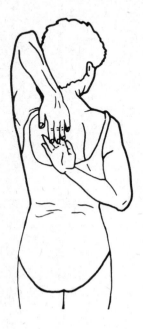

MENSTRUAL PAIN

Menstrual pain may involve nausea or headache, but the main symptom is abnormally painful uterine cramps, which at worst may be quite incapacitating. Such cramps may be caused by weakness in the uterine muscles or the abnormal position of the uterus, making the expulsion of menstrual blood difficult. Emotional factors and hormonal imbalance are other factors often mentioned in connection with menstrual pain, but leaving causes aside, shiatsu during the premenstrual days can make a noticeable improvement in how you feel during this time.

Women who are prone to menstrual pain often carry tension in the lower abdomen and back as well as shoulders and neck, particularly the back of the neck. Give special attention to your own or your partner's individual problem areas. Relieving tension in the lower abdomen and back during the premenstrual days will help prevent painful cramps, and giving regular shiatsu to these areas will correct hormone imbalances and condition the uterus.

1. Apply strong pressure to the medulla oblongata (page 18) with overlapping middle fingers.

2. Apply strong three-finger pressure to the upper-shoulder points.

3. Apply thumb pressure to the five lower-back points on either side of the spine, giving strong pressure to the last points.

4. Press the four points that run diagonally across each buttock, then the sternal points, especially the first.

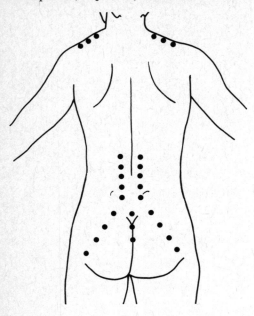

5. Give special attention to the Namikoshi points (page 18).

6. Press the lower abdominal and groin points, using palm pressure to both sides at once.

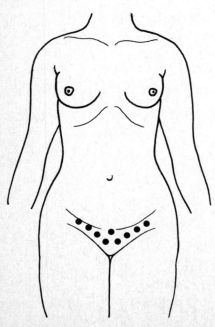

PREVENTING PROSTRATE TROUBLE

The prostate gland is part of the male reproductive system. It is about the size of a chestnut, is located below and to the rear of the bladder, and surrounds the basal section of the urethra. The fluid it secretes makes up part of the seminal fluid. Thus, when the prostate gland hypertrophies, or enlarges, not only urination but also sexual functioning is impeded. As hormonal secretion becomes unbalanced with age, the prostate gland increases in size, putting pressure on both the urethra and the spermatic duct. This condition is likely to worsen in the sixties and may lead to incontinence. First symptoms are irregular flow of urine, tiredness, and dry skin. Regular shiatsu can help prevent this condition and keep the body in good condition.

1. First, apply palm pressure to the point over the pubic bone.

2. Apply palm pressure to the groin points (see step 6 of the previous procedure).

3. Apply strong three-finger pressure on both sides of the base of the penis. Repeat several times. If you need to urinate, do so and then repeat.

4. Press the medulla oblongata (page 18) with overlapping middle fingers.

5. Clasp your hands behind your back and apply palm pressure to the kidneys with the heels of your hands.

6. Apply thumb pressure to the lower back and the sternum points.

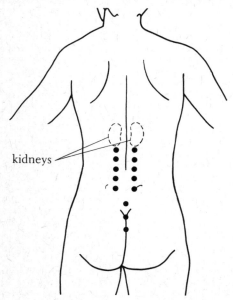

kidneys

7. Press the Namikoshi points (page 18).

8. Cup the testicles lightly in both palms. Squeeze and release thirty or forty times. This will stimulate hormone secretion and increase sexual vigor.

IMPROVING
APPEARANCE

Good looks and good health are so interrelated as to be virtually inseparable. No matter how physically attractive you may be, you cannot look your best when your eyes are puffy and bleary from too little sleep, when your posture is bad from poor muscle tone, or when your expression and disposition are sour because you have indigestion. The magic of cosmetics can work marvelous deceptions but touches only the surface. The kind of appeal that radiates from a strong, healthy body and a clear, balanced mind is deep and long-lasting. The role of shiatsu is to help you achieve such a foundation. This chapter will deal with the two aspects of physical appearance many people worry most about, skin care and losing weight.

SKIN CARE

Having smooth, attractive skin is not simply a matter of applying external treatment. Beautiful skin is created from the inside. It is a natural reflection of a radiantly healthy body and mind.

The greater part of skin care is attention to one's general health. Among the causes of skin problems are constipation and indigestion, so it is important to maintain normal functioning of the digestive organs. Lack of exercise, excess weight, emotional upsets, and irregular eating and sleeping habits can also contribute to skin problems. When the functioning of the skin is poor, it becomes pale, rough-textured, dry, dull, spotted, and wrinkled.

Shiatsu is not just a matter of giving temporary stimulation to the skin by patting or massaging, but of giving gradual, steady finger pressure to specific points on the body surface. This pressure penetrates deep into the muscles, relaxing tension and releasing pressure on the blood vessels, lymph glands, and nerves. In shiatsu the intensity of pressure is varied according to the degree of muscle stiffness in each area, thus conditioning the whole body. Full-body shiatsu activates the functioning of the skin, stimulates tissue regeneration and blood circulation, and helps to maintain a fresh, moist, smooth complexion.

Proper hormone secretion is most important to the skin. Shiatsu to the adrenal and thyroid glands is particularly helpful. The adrenal glands secrete about sixty types of hormones.

Proper circulation is also important to the skin, particularly to the hands. If you have trouble with dry, chapped, cracked, or cold hands, give yourself regular shiatsu to improve the circulation to your hands and restore the regenerative function of the skin.

1. First apply thumb pressure to points along the front of the neck, first left, then right. This stimulates blood flow to the head, giving good color to the complexion as well as clearing away grogginess. Between the third and fourth points is the thyroid gland, which gives glossiness to the complexion.

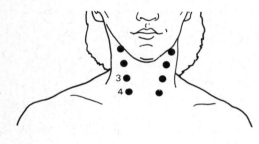

2. Apply three-finger pressure to the points on each side of the neck.

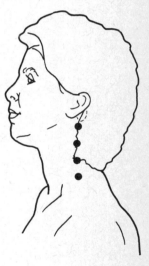

3. Press the points on each side of the back of the neck, then the upper-shoulder points—left, then right—for five seconds each.

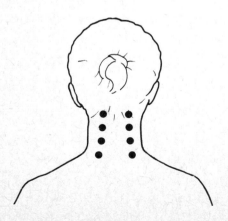

4. Next, give shiatsu to the face. Apply three-finger pressure to the forehead, the sides of the nose (use overlapping middle/index finger pressure here), the edges of the cheekbones, the side of the mouth, and the upper and lower eye sockets. Give special attention, gradually increasing pressure, to any areas where the skin is dry, wrinkled, or rough.

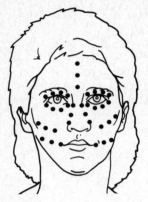

5. Press the temple points using three-finger pressure. Shiatsu to these points will keep the skin pliant and prevent crow's-feet.

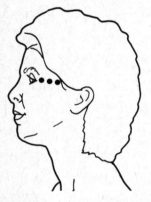

6. Press the adrenal glands on either side of the backbone, at the top of the kidneys (the third lower-back points, page 29). For self-shiatsu, clasp your hands behind your back and press with your palms.

7. If you are prone to constipation, press the abdominal points.

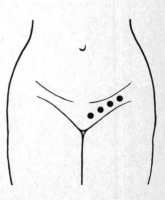

8. For improving circulation to the hands, press the arm and hand points (pages 41–46).

SLIMMING AND TONING

If you are concerned with losing weight and improving muscle tone, you probably already have an exercise program of some kind. Try doing self-shiatsu along with your warm-ups or stretching before vigorous exercise, and afterward as you relax and take a bath or shower.

■ Neck

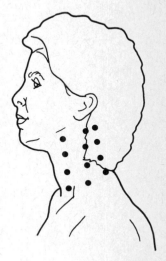

Traditional Japanese standards of beauty place great emphasis on the neck, particularly the lines of the nape as it emerges from the collar of the kimono. Modern-day Western standards are rather different, but nonetheless, neither a tense, stringy neck nor a flabby neck is very attractive. A common sign of aging is the sagging posture and protruding chin resulting from loss of elasticity in the neck muscles.

Shiatsu to the neck muscles, particularly to the points on the front of the neck along the carotid artery and the vagus nerve, and on the back of the neck, is crucial for good health as well as appearance. It is particularly beneficial in treating fatigue and insomnia, which are detrimental to anyone's appearance. Follow the instructions for shiatsu to the neck (page 22). Try to give yourself this shiatsu when you wake up in the morning, before you go to bed, and while relaxing in a hot bath.

■ Breasts

In order to keep the breasts both healthy and shapely, it is important to release tension in the chest, have good posture, and maintain proper hormone secretion. Shiatsu certainly cannot produce dramatic changes in breast size, but regular shiatsu to the breasts can improve muscle tone, thus increasing firmness and uplift and preventing sagging.

1. First, to maintain proper hormone secretion, press the points on the front of the neck, on either side of the thyroid gland.

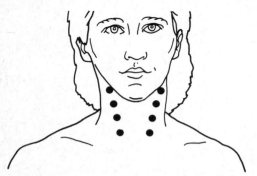

2. Press the medulla oblongata (page 18) with overlapping middle fingers.

3. Press the third lower-back points (page 29), first with palm pressure, then with thumb pressure.

4. Use the fingers of both hands simultaneously to press the points between the ribs, three rows of four points on each side, working around the breasts. Work outward from the breastbone. Repeat twice.

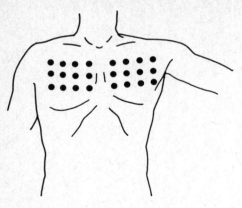

5. Place both palms under your armpits and press inward, squeezing the breasts together. Repeat twice.

6. Press the side of the left breast with the base of the palms and link fingers at the front. Apply counterclockwise circular pressure ten times. Then grasp the base of the nipple gently between thumb and forefinger and lift up. Repeat the circular pressure. Repeat the same procedure for the right breast, in a clockwise motion.

■ Waist

When you are working on slimming the waist, a combination of shiatsu and stretching is helpful.

1. Apply thumb pressure to the points on each side of the back along the upper edge of the hipbone.

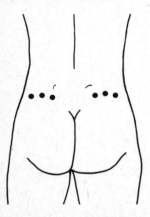

2. Put both hands on your hips and, without moving your feet, twist as far as possible to the right, hold for five seconds, then twist to the left and hold. Do five times.

3. With hands in the same position, squeeze the waist ten times.

■ Abdomen

This shiatsu is good for the sagging abdominal muscles that come with aging, childbirth, or excess weight.

1. First, apply three-finger pressure to the three points on each side of the navel, working inward.

2. Next, work outward from the bladder area, applying three-finger pressure for five seconds to the two sets of points on the lower abdomen.

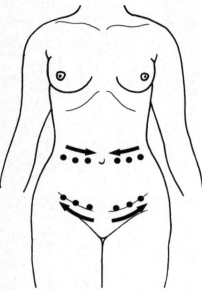

3. Place your palms at your sides just above the hip bones, level with the points in step 2. Apply palm pressure while sliding your hands quickly forward until the palms meet in front of the navel. Do five times.

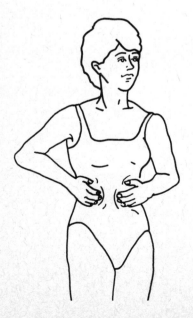

■ Hips

The following simple sequence will help reduce excess flesh and tone the muscles of the hip area.

1. Apply three-finger pressure to the points on each side of the crest of the hipbone.

2. Press the points running diagonally across the buttocks.

3. Apply three-finger pressure to the points directly beneath the buttocks and lift up for three seconds.

4. Apply suction pressure again to the buttocks with a rolling motion of the knuckles of both fists.

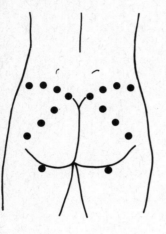

■ Legs

Often when the legs appear heavy and swollen, the cause is not simply excess weight but poor circulation. Begin shiatsu for the legs by applying overlapping-palm pressure to the three points of the groin. This stimulates blood flow to the legs. Then follow the procedure for shiatsu for the legs and feet given on pages 30–33 and 36–41. This will relieve swelling, fatigue, and cold feet, and also improve coordination.

SHIATSU AND STRETCHING

Shiatsu releases muscle tension and stiffness, increases flexibility, and relieves fatigue. Stretching extends the muscles, improves circulation, and gives greater muscular strength and resilience. When the two are combined, they complement and reinforce each other, and the results are that much more beneficial. Basically, shiatsu is used here to relax and limber tired muscles; then stretching can increase strength and flexibility. Stretching will also give the joints improved range and ease of motion. Stretching should be performed slowly and be coordinated with breathing. The extended position should be held for the given time, then released.

No special equipment or locale is required to do these exercises. Three minutes here and five minutes there—when you think of it or feel a little tired or stiff—can be quite helpful. If you can't set aside a special time and place when you can really concentrate, at least take a few minutes after a bath or shower, before bed, or during a break from work to fit a few minutes of shiatsu stretching into your daily schedule.

The instructions here are given for each section of the body. As you learn the techniques, you may want to practice one or two sections a day on a rotating schedule. It will gradually become a natural part of your daily life to pay attention to the areas where fatigue and tension have accumulated.

NOTE: Unless otherwise stated, do the left side, then the right, for each step.

FACE

1. Apply three-finger pressure to the upper and then lower eye-socket points, working outward. Then, still using three-finger pressure, slide the fingers slowly over the same points, pulling the skin outward. When you reach the last point, hold for ten seconds and release. Do both sides simultaneously for steps 1 through 4.

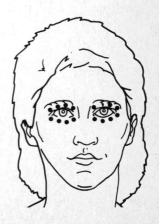

2. Apply three-finger pressure to the temples, then "pull" the skin as in step 1.

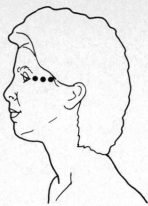

3. Apply overlapping middle/index-finger pressure to the points at the sides of the nose. Then pull the skin along the same points for ten seconds.

4. Apply three-finger pressure to the forehead, working from the center outward; then move the fingers slowly over the same points, stretching the skin. Follow the same procedure for the points at the sides of the mouth.

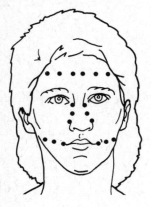

NECK

1. Apply thumb pressure to the left side of the neck first, then to the right. Make sure you do only one side at a time.

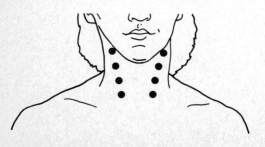

2. Place both hands under your jaw and tilt your head backward to stretch the skin at the front of the neck. Hold for ten seconds and release.

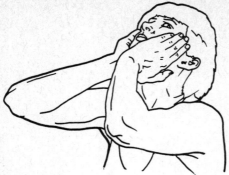

3. Apply three-finger pressure to both sides of the neck at the same time.

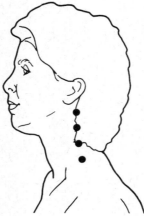

4. With your right hand, pull your head to the right, stretching the left side of the neck. Hold for ten seconds. Repeat with the left side, using the left hand.

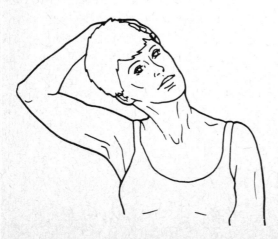

5. Apply three-finger pressure to both sides of the back of the neck at the same time.

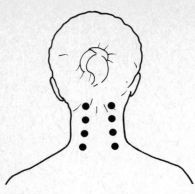

6. Clasp your hands behind your neck and bend your neck backward. Hold for ten seconds, then release.

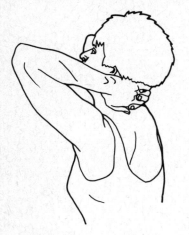

SHOULDERS AND ARMS

1. Apply three-finger pressure to the upper shoulder, then to the groove between the shoulder and the chest.

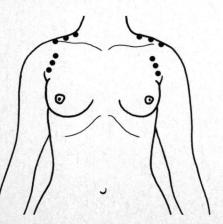

2. Reach under your left arm with your right hand and apply three-finger pressure to the three rows of three points along the muscles which connect the shoulder blade and the base of the arm.

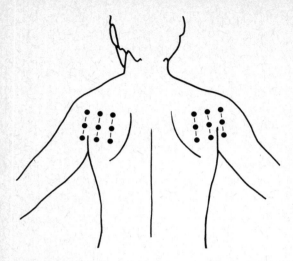

3. Apply three-finger pressure to the center row of shoulder points, then use opposing thumb and fingers to press the two outer rows simultaneously.

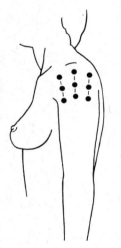

4. Use opposing thumb and fingers to press the top and underside of the arm simultaneously.

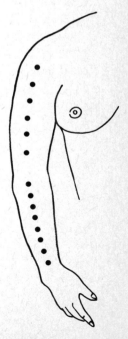

5. Slowly rotate your shoulders in a circular motion ten times forward, then ten times backward.

6. Place your right hand on your left elbow and reach down your back with your left hand as far as you can. Hold the position for ten seconds, then release.

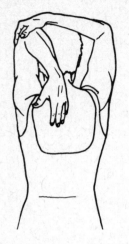

7. Reach behind your back with your left hand and push up on your arm with your right hand. Hold for ten seconds, then release.

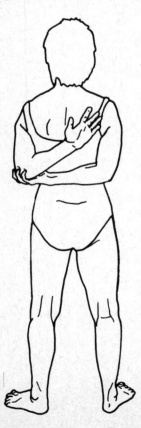

8. Try to touch or clasp your hands behind your back with one elbow up and one down. Hold for ten seconds, then release.

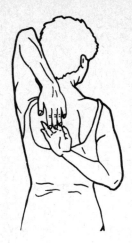

9. Clasp your hands, palms out, and extend your arms straight in front of you. Hold this position for ten seconds, then release. Clasp your hands above your head and repeat, then behind your back, palms inward.

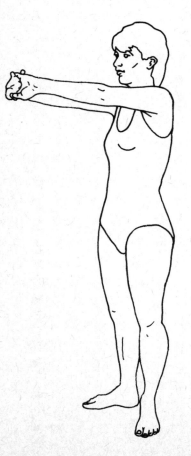

HANDS

1. Use opposing thumb and fingers to press the three rows on the top and bottom of the wrist at the same time. Begin with the row nearest the thumb and work toward the elbow.

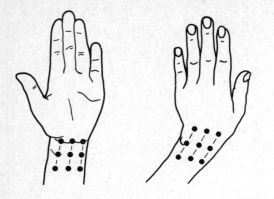

2. Apply thumb pressure to the four rows on the palm of the hand, then to the corresponding points on the back of the hand. Begin with the row nearest the thumb and work toward the fingers.

3. Use your thumb and forefinger to press the finger and thumb points. After pressing each finger, pull it straight outward.

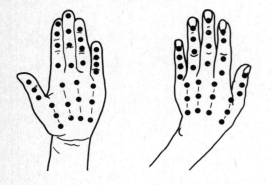

4. Put the fingertips of both hands together and extend the fingers apart as far as possible. In this open position, rotate the hands forward and backward ten times. Then bend each wrist backward at a right angle, alternating left and right, ten times.

5. Extend your arms in front of you and bring your fingertips together, release, then swing your arms behind you and bring your fingertips together again. Do five times.

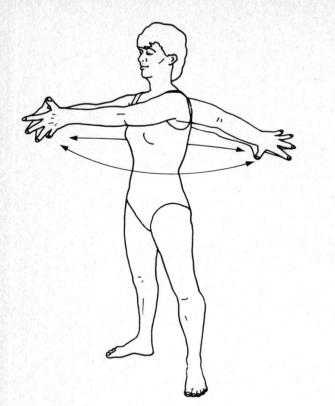

BACK

1. Apply three-finger pressure to the top three points on either side of the spine, first using your right hand for the left side, then your left hand for the right side.

2. Apply thumb pressure to the ten points on both sides of the spine simultaneously, working down from the bottom of the shoulder blades.

3. Sit on a stool or lean against a wall, clasp your hands behind your neck, and bend forward and then straighten up. Repeat ten times.

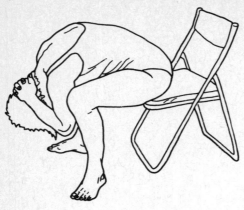

LEGS AND FEET

1. Apply overlapping-thumb pressure to the top and inside of the thigh. Then apply two-thumb pressure to the outside of the thigh. Work toward the feet.

2. Apply thumb pressure to the points around the kneecap.

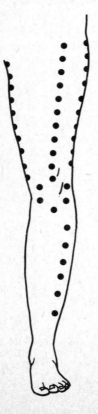

3. Grasp the toes of your left foot in your right hand; then, with your thumb, press first the ankle points, then the instep.

4. Support the ankle with your right hand and, with your left thumb and index finger, press the toe points.

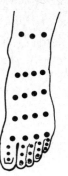

5. Apply three-finger pressure with both hands to the underside of the thigh. Then use overlapping-thumb pressure on the back of the knee.

6. Continue down the points on the underside of the calf, then press the sides of the calf with opposing thumb and fingers.

7. Apply two-thumb pressure to the sole of the foot.

8. To stretch the back of the leg, rest your foot on the back of a chair. Pull back on your toes. Hold for ten seconds, then release.

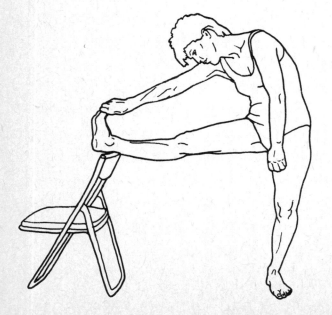

9. To stretch the front of the leg, brace yourself with your left hand against a wall and bend your left leg back. Grab the foot by the ankle and pull up. Hold for ten seconds, then release.

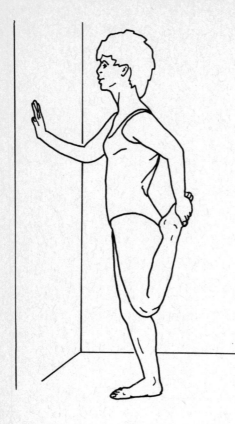

10. Bend the foot forward, then backward, holding for ten seconds in each position.

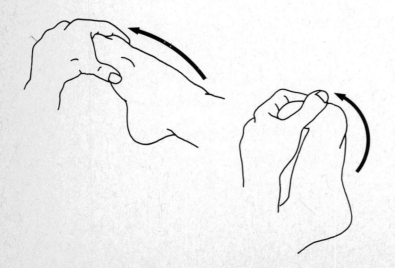

CHEST

1. Use index, middle, and ring fingers to press three rows at a time. Do both sides simultaneously, working outward. For women, work around the breasts.

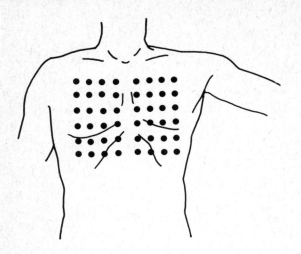

2. Clasp your hands behind your back. Extend your arms diagonally behind you, tilt your head back, and expand your chest. Hold for ten seconds, then relax.

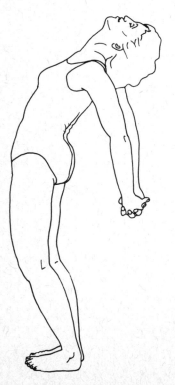

ABDOMEN

1. Apply palm pressure with both hands to the two central rows. Repeat on the left side and then the right.

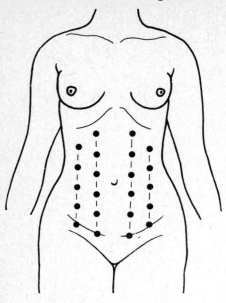

2. Give the same pressure to the ten-point series.

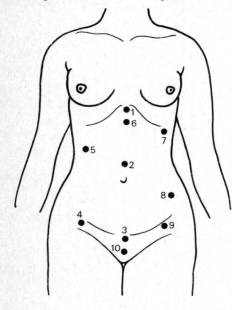

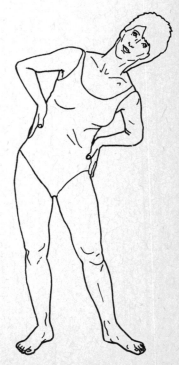

3. Place your hands at your sides as shown. Bend to the right and to the left, holding for ten seconds each time.

4. Place your left hand over your navel and your right hand on your lower back. Twist to the right (in the direction in which the hand over the navel is pointing) and hold for ten seconds. Reverse your hands and twist to the left.

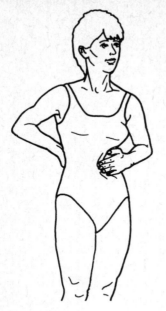

5. Bracing yourself as shown, bend backward. Hold the position for ten seconds, then straighten up.

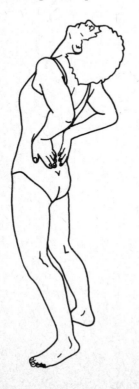

SHIATSU
FOR
CHILDREN

Spending time with your child by giving him shiatsu, or doing shiatsu together, is a wonderful way to help him build a strong, healthy body while teaching him good habits at the same time. Shiatsu time should be fun and pleasant for the child, so avoid giving him shiatsu when he is tired, ill, or hungry or has just eaten. If you give your child shiatsu regularly, you will become aware of slight changes in condition from day to day and be able to give special attention where it is needed.

The procedures here are for preschool-age children, but even infants as young as one month can benefit from shiatsu. (For a discussion about older children, see the last paragraph.) While changing the baby's diaper or bathing him, stroke his body gently. A baby is so sensitive that a very light touch is sufficient. Use your index or middle finger alone, or both held in a V-position, or your palm, and always be sure your hands are warm. Long sessions are too much for a baby; short periods on a regular basis are most effective. Also, do not give shiatsu when the baby is tired or feverish. Sleep is what he needs most then.

The preschool years are most important for building a strong constitution and resistance to disease. If your child has health problems, such as asthma, rather than label him a sickly child, treat him with love and patience. Give him shiatsu often and make sure he gets plenty of fresh air, exercise, and good food. Give him confidence that he can become strong and healthy.

When giving shiatsu to small children, make sure your hands are warm, and your fingernails trimmed. Gentle stroking and palm pressure are what you will use most. When an exercise calls for finger pressure, make sure you press gently; strong finger pressure is unpleasant for children.

Let your hands teach you about your child's body. Find the correct points and adjust the type, degree, and duration of pressure according to the condition of the area you are working on. Shiatsu time does not have to be a serious, forced activity. Let your child talk about friends, preschool, or day care; make it a time for relaxed communication.

For older children, shiatsu is a way to maintain good health, relieve stress from school, prevent sports injuries, and encourage good health-care habits. Practicing shiatsu with your child will help you keep in touch with him despite busy schedules and be aware of any problems in their early stages. As your child grows older, you may adjust your shiatsu techniques accordingly, always making sure that the shiatsu is pleasant for the child. Many of the procedures given in other sections of this book are also appropriate for older children.

NOTE: In some areas, such as the back of the neck, back, and abdomen, fewer points are shown than for an adult's body. This simply reflects the difference in proportion between an adult's hand and a child's body.

COUGHING

Coughing occurs with the inflammation of the throat and windpipe that accompanies the common cold, as well as with more serious ailments like asthma, whooping cough, and tuberculosis. Coughing may be dry and hacking, ticklish and shallow, or deep and wrenching, but when it continues it is painful and exhausting. Because coughing deprives the child of the sleep he needs so much to get well, it is important to give prompt shiatsu treatment to bring relief. However, coughing is only a symptom, and bringing temporary relief is not enough. The cause must also be determined. If you suspect your child's cough is more than a common cold, be sure to seek medical help promptly.

1. The sternocleidomastoid muscle extends diagonally from behind the ear, past the Adam's apple, to the collarbone. When this muscle is tight, it presses on the windpipe and aggravates coughing. Shiatsu to the front neck points, which run along this muscle, will help to bring relief. However, because a major artery runs beneath these points, it is dangerous to press them very strongly in small children. Instead of pressing, stroke gently downward with your thumb or with three fingers. Repeat several times.

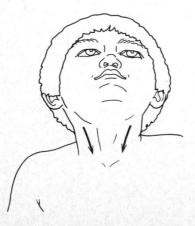

2. Stroke one side of the chest from the center outward while supporting the back with your free hand. Repeat for the other side. This will also relax the tension around the windpipe and make breathing easier.

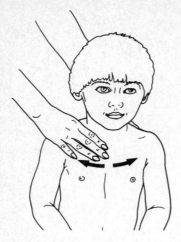

3. Supporting the head with your left hand, grasp the back of the neck between your thumb and three fingers and press for three seconds. At the same time, tilt the head backward slightly to stretch the front neck muscles.

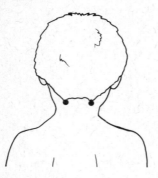

4. Have the child bend his head backward while at the same time expanding the chest by breathing in deeply.

ASTHMA

Asthma, an allergic ailment characterized by attacks of wheezing and labored breathing, is becoming more and more common in children. When the attack passes, the child quickly returns to normal. Children who have been prone to respiratory congestion as infants often begin to have asthmatic attacks when they enter early childhood. Asthma is most often seen in children between two and ten. In such cases, the child is usually constitutionally predisposed to asthma, but allergic reactions may be triggered by air pollution, pollen, household dust or mold, certain foods, or the fur of household pets. Thus, it may be necessary to remove such sources of trouble by keeping a dust-free house, getting rid of pets, or restricting certain foods.

However, a child who suffers from asthma is not necessarily condemned to an asthmatic adulthood. It is possible to help a child break free of asthma by making sure he gets enough exercise, fresh air, and sunshine. Keep his skin healthy by giving frequent rubdowns with a dry towel. And give him shiatsu regularly to improve his general physical condition. Don't wait until the asthma attacks come, but try to establish the discipline of giving him shiatsu twice daily, morning and evening. The treatment of childhood asthma can be a long struggle, but with patience and love you can help your child achieve good health.

The following procedure should also bring substantial relief in case of an asthmatic attack.

1. Follow steps 1 and 2 of the procedure for Coughing (page 123).

2. An asthmatic child will usually have an abnormally narrow space between the shoulder blades and the spine. Have the child lie on his right side and apply overlapping-thumb pressure to the upper-shoulder point. Then gently press the upper-back points on the left side. Repeat for the right side. Then have the child lie on his stomach and press both sets of back points with your thumbs simultaneously.

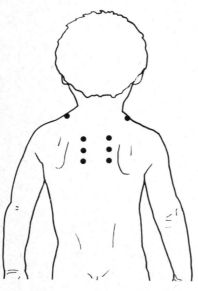

3. Have the child sit on the floor or on a stool. Grasp both shoulders from the side and lift them up, then let them drop naturally. Do ten times. Then rotate the shoulders ten times forward and ten times backward. This will relax both the back and chest muscles.

4. After making sure that your hands are warm, place your palms, with fingertips together, on the upper part of the child's chest. Stroke outward along the muscles between the ribs. Repeat twice, moving your hands slightly lower on the chest each time.

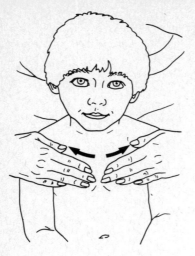

5. Place both palms lightly on the chest, fingers pointing down. Press with a circular movement, repeating several times. Next, stroke down the chest twice. Then you may press the chest once more and hold for about five seconds.

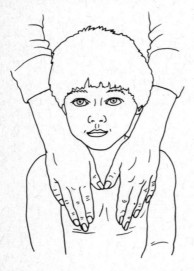

6. To finish, have the child lie on his back and place your palm on the solar plexus (page 19). In children who have been coughing, it will be stiff and tender. Press lightly as the child exhales. Repeat several times.

NASAL CONGESTION

Congestion and a runny nose are enough to make most adults miserable. Children, too, become irritable, impatient, and dull-witted when they have a cold. Also, in cases of sinusitis, the nasal mucous is thickened, causing headache and eye fatigue and also leading to sleeplessness and dulling of the memory and mental faculties. Early shiatsu can bring relief and speed recovery.

1. First, press the points on both sides of the nose simultaneously using overlapping index/middle fingers or just index fingers.

2. Apply overlapping-thumb pressure to the forehead points. The lowest point, between the eyebrows, is particularly effective when the sinuses are congested.

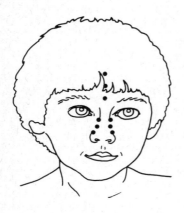

3. Press each point around the eye sockets slowly and gently using thumb pressure, and along the edges of the cheekbones using three-finger pressure.

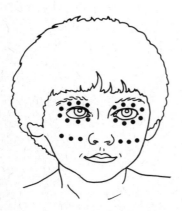

4. Apply three-finger pressure to the temple points.

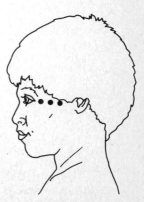

5. Stroke down the points on the front of the neck—left, then right—using your thumb or three fingers. Do about five times.

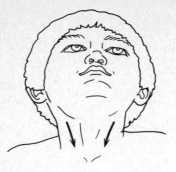

6. Press the back of the neck, grasping with your thumb and fingers. Be careful not to press too strongly.

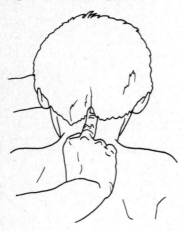

7. Have the child bend his neck forward and back and sideways to stretch the neck muscles.

STOMACHACHE

When children complain of a stomachache, the pain may or may not be accompanied by diarrhea, or it may simply go away after a bowel movement. It may be caused by eating or drinking too much, by a chill in the abdomen, a cold, or nervous upset. Whatever the cause, the functioning of the digestive system is weakened and digestion is impaired. Particularly diarrhea, if left untreated, may lead to dehydration and lowered resistance due to lack of nutrition. In such cases it is important to see that the child gets plenty of fluids and recovers quickly. Stomachache may sometimes be a symptom of an infectious disease. If it is accompanied by high fever or you suspect it is more than a simple cold or digestive irregularity, be sure to seek prompt medical diagnosis.

In cases of stomachache or diarrhea, the solar plexus will feel stiff and chilled because of poor blood flow to the abdominal organs. The back muscles will also be stiff. Shiatsu to these areas stimulates blood flow and restores normal functioning.

1. Have the child lie either on his side or his stomach. Apply thumb pressure to the back points for three seconds each, one side at a time. Repeat twice.

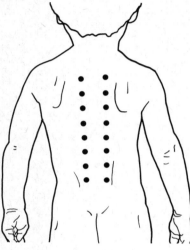

2. In cases of diarrhea, apply thumb pressure to both Namikoshi points (page 18) simultaneously for five seconds. Repeat twice. Be careful not to press too hard.

3. Have the child turn onto his back. Apply palm pressure to the abdominal points. Then move your palm clockwise in a full circle, as though you are warming the abdomen with your palm. Be sure to synchronize the pressure with the child's breathing, pressing as the child exhales.

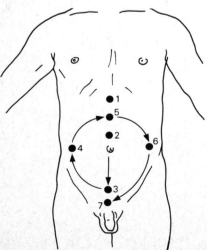

POOR APPETITE

Although appetites vary greatly, obviously a child needs a good appetite to grow and thrive. If your child seems to lose his appetite for no apparent reason, consider whether he is getting enough exercise or is irritable for some reason. Also stop and think whether you are nagging him constantly about not eating or his manners and behavior during meals.

Children need plenty of exercise, as much of it as possible outdoors. They also need a relaxed, pleasant atmosphere at mealtime. Children also love a change of routine, like eating outdoors, some colorful and interesting new tableware, or a savory new meal.

A child with sluggish digestion and a poor appetite will generally have stiffness in the back and solar plexus. Shiatsu to these areas will stimulate the digestive organs and thus improve the appetite.

1. Have the child lie on his back. Apply palm pressure slowly to the abdominal points above the navel, moving the hand slightly lower each time.

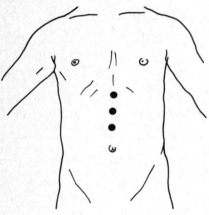

2. Have the child turn onto his stomach and work down the back points to the area over the stomach, using thumb pressure to both sides at once. Repeat three times.

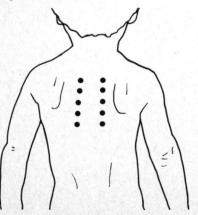

3. Have the child sit on the floor with legs extended. Kneel behind him and brace his back against your thigh. Grasp his lower arms near the wrists and pull upward and back. Repeat several times. This also stimulates the back and solar plexus.

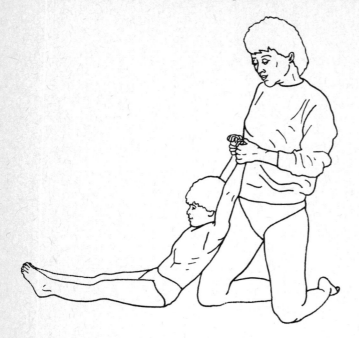

LISTLESSNESS

What do you do with a child who is tired and listless? His movements are slow; his voice is expressionless. He lies on the floor watching television and has no enthusiasm or energy. Of course, if there is some specific physical problem, it must have special attention. But when there is no particular cause for the child's lethargic state, he needs both mental and physical stimulation. Rather than the standard parental refrain: "What's wrong with you? Don't just mope around the house, go out and play," try a few minutes of shiatsu.

1. First, feel and press the child's body to check for stiffness in the back or legs, or abnormal curvature of the spine. Poor posture can be a cause of tiredness.

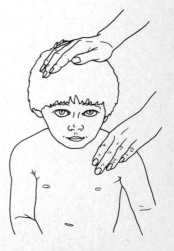

2. Have the child sit on the floor or in a chair. Standing behind the chair, place your left hand on your child's left shoulder and, with your right hand, apply slow, steady pressure to the crown of the head for three to five seconds. Repeat several times. In small children, whose skulls are not yet fully developed, it is better not to use thumb pressure.

3. Support the forehead with your left hand and, with your right thumb or middle finger, press the medulla oblongata (page 18), in the direction of the point between the eyebrows, for five seconds. Repeat several times.

4. Now that you have given shiatsu to the head, move on to the extremities. First, apply strong two-thumb pressure to the arch point on the sole of the foot. Then press the end of each toe top and bottom with thumb and index finger, pulling gently. Repeat for the other foot.

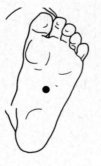

5. Apply strong pressure to the center of the palm of the left hand with overlapping thumbs. Then press and pull each finger in the same manner as the toes. Repeat for the other hand.

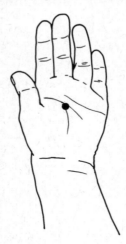

6. Fatigue often shows up as stiffness in the back. Have the child lie on his stomach. Rub down the back from between the shoulder blades to the hips. Repeat several times. Then apply thumb pressure to both Namikoshi points (page 18) at the same time.

POOR EYESIGHT

Today's urban environment provides more and more sources of eyestrain, even for small children. Some children spend hours in front of a television or computer screen. Although it is so important, it is easy to forget to rest the eyes as soon as they become tired. This you can teach your child best by example.

If eye care is neglected in small children, temporary vision problems can become permanent. Good eye-care habits are best established and problems corrected before the child reaches school age. You can catch early signs of eye trouble by observing your child. Do you often notice him bleary-eyed or squinting? When he looks at books, does he have good posture and proper light? Shiatsu to relieve eyestrain will help to improve your child's vision and teach him good habits.

1. When the eyes are tired, the shoulders become stiff and the neck difficult to bend backward. The head slumps forward as the child strains to see. To release this shoulder tension, have the child lie on his stomach, then press the neck points, shoulder points, and the upper-back points between the shoulder blades, using thumb pressure to both sides at once.

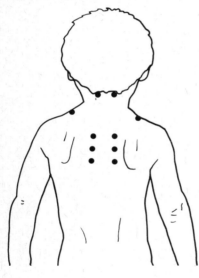

2. Have the child sit on the floor. Kneel behind him and brace his back against your thigh. Grasp his lower arms near the wrists and pull slowly up and back. Repeat several times.

3. Have the child lie on his back for shiatsu to the eye area. Apply light thumb pressure to the eight points around the edges of the eye sockets, the points just above the center of each eyebrow, and the temples.

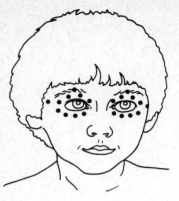

MOTION SICKNESS

Headache and nausea brought on by the motion of cars, buses, boats, and in extreme cases even trains or playground swings, often spoils an outing for all of the participants. Generally, people prone to motion sickness tend to be nervous, sensitive to smells, and have weak stomachs. Once a child has experienced motion sickness, he may be prone to self-suggestion and be even more likely to get sick. Likewise, if you are overanxious, it will only have a negative effect on the child. Lack of sleep and an empty stomach will also increase the likelihood of motion sickness, so make sure your child is well rested and fed before a trip. During the trip, open a window to let fresh air into the vehicle. Shiatsu to release tension is a good preventive measure.

1. First, press the sides of the neck. Tension here increases the pressure of lymphatic fluid in the inner ear, disturbing the sense of balance and causing dizziness. Supporting the forehead with your left hand, grasp the sides of the neck with your thumb and fingers just below the bony projection of the skull behind the ears and press for three seconds. Repeat several times.

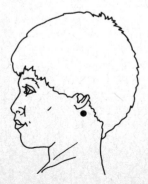

2. Press the medulla oblongata (page 18) with your middle finger for five seconds. Repeat twice. Also, press the shoulders and upper back.

Shiatsu to the neck points above, particularly the points just behind the earlobes, is helpful when a child begins to feel nauseous while traveling. An older child may be taught to use self-shiatsu when he feels sick.

3. Have the child lie on his back and apply gentle palm pressure to the abdominal points, coordinating the pressure with the child's breathing. Give particular attention to the solar plexus (points 1, 2, and 5). Tension here produces the feeling of nausea.

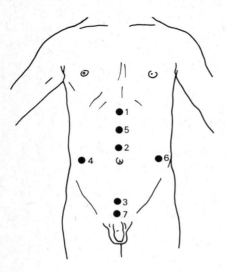

OVERSENSITIVITY

Oversensitive children are so sensitive to events and people around them that they are prone to nervous exhaustion. This may lead to problems such as bed-wetting or extreme fastidiousness. When you give shiatsu to such a child, do it in a warm, relaxed atmosphere, letting him chat naturally. When the child's nerves are strained, his fingers will be chilly. Simply holding his hands in yours to warm them will help to calm him. Shiatsu to the hands soothes the nerves by stimulating circulation to the head.

1. Press the finger points, grasping the finger between thumb and forefinger and pulling gently.

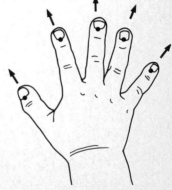

2. Give strong pressure to the center of the palm with overlapping thumbs for three to five seconds. Repeat twice.

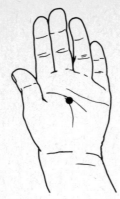

3. Press the medulla oblongata (page 18) with your middle finger for five seconds. Repeat twice.

4. Apply palm pressure to the solar plexus (page 19) three to five times.

5. Have the child hold his hands apart as though to clap them, with fingers spread. He then alternates pressing his fingertips together and pulling his hands apart. Try adding rhythm with a song or rhyme.

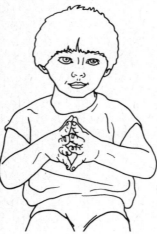

BED-WETTING

When urine accumulates in the bladder, a signal is sent to the brain, which then orders the bladder muscles to contract, thus causing urination. This mechanism does not develop completely until about the age of three, but after one year the amount of urine produced at night decreases naturally, and between the ages of two to four most children sleep through the night without urinating. A pituitary hormone is responsible for the reduction of urine production at night. Children who have insufficient secretion of this hormone may reach age five or six with no decrease in night urine, and be prone to chronic bed-wetting. Most cases of bed-wetting are of this type, but other physiological or psychological factors may be involved.

In any case, your own irritation and uneasiness will only increase the child's anxiety and bring negative results. Try not to lose your patience, do not scold, and do not wake the child in the night to make him urinate. Remain calm and refrain from saying or doing things that may humiliate the child and cause him to lose confidence. Speak to him soothingly and give him the warmth of your touch with shiatsu.

1. To regulate the connection between the brain and the bladder, support the forehead with your left hand and press the medulla oblongata (page 18) with your right middle finger for five seconds. Repeat twice.

2. Next, press the back points, giving particular attention to the lower back and the sacrum.

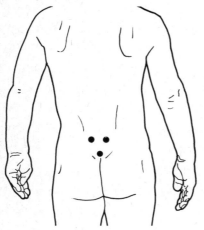

3. Apply thumb pressure to both Namikoshi points (page 18) at once for five seconds. Repeat twice.

4. Apply palm pressure to the abdominal points, giving particular attention to the area over the bladder (point 7).

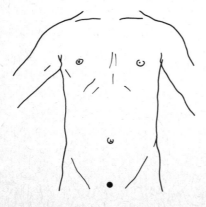

5. Apply thumb or three-finger pressure to the groin points.

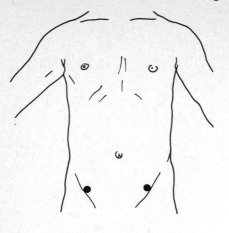

6. You may also give shiatsu to the legs and feet, particularly to the soles of the feet.

THUMB-SUCKING, NAIL-BITING

When a three- or four-year-old child still sucks his thumb or bites his nails, we are apt to say something like "He doesn't know what to do with himself" or "He's not interested in anything." However, this so-called apathy can be considered a kind of nervousness. It does no good to scold the child. You must deal with the basic question of how to stimulate his curiosity and will-power. He needs a place and means to express his creativity. Is he getting enough playtime, exercise, time with family and friends? Or enough chances to sing, paint, or read aloud? The following points are particularly good for energizing an apathetic child. Doing shiatsu together not only helps effect a cure but also can be a pleasant, relaxed time when he can talk about his friends and activities at day care or school.

1. Have the child lie on his back. Apply overlapping-thumb pressure to the point between the eyebrows for three seconds. Repeat twice.

2. With your forefingers, press the first point on the upper inside of the eye socket, left and right simultaneously, then the three points on each side of the nose. Repeat twice.

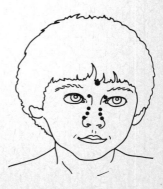

3. Have the child sit up. Steadying his left shoulder with your left hand, apply palm pressure to the crown of the head for three seconds, three times. Then apply palm pressure to both sides of the head at once, three times.

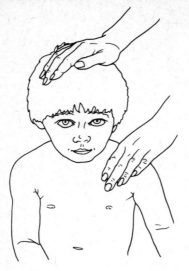

ABOUT THE AUTHOR

Toru Namikoshi, director of the Japan Shiatsu College, is the leading practitioner of shiatsu in Japan. He travels extensively to lecture and conduct seminars on the subject. He is the author of several books on the art of shiatsu including the major technical manual for students and medical specialists *The Complete Book of Shiatsu Therapy*. His books have found wide acceptance and have been translated into French, German, Italian, Spanish, Dutch and even Danish. The present volume is his most comprehensive and up-to-date work for the layman.

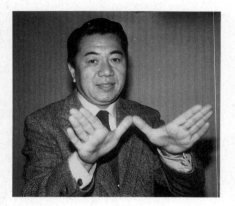